The Fainting Phenomenon

UNDERSTANDING WHY PEOPLE FAINT
AND WHAT TO DO ABOUT IT

To Barbara Straus MD. Physician, wife, mother and soul mate; and to Helen and Alex never-ending sources of pride and joy; and to Paul B. Grubb ... may his memory be for a blessing.

The Fainting Phenomenon

UNDERSTANDING WHY PEOPLE FAINT AND WHAT TO DO ABOUT IT

Second Edition

Blair P. Grubb, MD
Professor of Medicine and Pediatrics
Director, Cardiac Electrophysiology Section and
Clinical Autonomic Disorders Center
University Medical Center
Health Science Campus
University of Toledo School of Medicine
Toledo, Ohio, USA

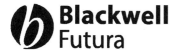

Blackwell
Futura

© 2001 Futura Publishing Company, Inc., New York
© 2007 Blair P. Grubb
Published by Blackwell Publishing
Blackwell Futura is an imprint of Blackwell Publishing

Blackwell Publishing Inc., 350 Main Street, Malden, Massachusetts 02148-5020, USA
Blackwell Publishing Ltd, 9600 Garsington Road, Oxford OX4 2DQ, UK
Blackwell Science Asia Pty Ltd, 550 Swanston Street, Carlton, Victoria 3053, Australia

First published 2001
Second edition 2007

1   2007

ISBN: 978-1-4051-4841-2

Library of Congress Cataloging-in-Publication Data

Grubb, Blair P.
    The fainting phenomenon : understanding why people faint and what to do about it/
by Blair P. Grubb. – 2nd ed.
        p.   cm.
    Includes bibliographical references and index.
    ISBN-13: 978-1-4051-4841-2
    ISBN-10: 1-4051-4841-1
1.   Syncope (pathology) – popular works.   I.   Title.

    RB150. S9G78 2007
    616′.047–dc22

                                                                        2006025823

A catalogue record for this title is available from the British Library

Acquisitions: Gina Almond
Development: Beckie Brand
Set in 9.5/12 Palatino by TechBooks, India
Printed and bound in Singapore by Markono Print Media Pte Ltd

For further information on Blackwell Publishing, visit our website:
www.blackwellcardiology.com

The publisher's policy is to use permanent paper from mills that operate a sustainable forestry
policy, and which has been manufactured from pulp processed using acid-free and elementary
chlorine-free practices. Furthermore, the publisher ensures that the text paper and cover board
used have met acceptable environmental accreditation standards.

Contents

About the author

Blair P. Grubb, MD, is a Professor of Medicine and Pediatrics at the University of Toledo, School of Medicine, in Toledo, OH. A native of Baltimore, MD, Dr Grubb joined the University's faculty in 1988, after completing training in cardiovascular disease and electrophysiology at the Pennsylvania State University. He has been involved in research into the causes of fainting and autonomic nervous system disorders since 1988.

Dr Grubb has written over 160 scientific papers and is the coeditor of a textbook for physicians on fainting (*Syncope: Mechanisms and Management.* Blackwell Publishing Ltd., 2005). He received the University of Maryland's Distinguished Alumnus Award in 1994 and the Medical College's Dean's Award for Teaching Excellence in 1996, the Legacy of Achievement Award from the Northwest Ohio American Heart Association in 2001, and the Physician of the Year Award from the National Dysautonomia Research Foundation in 2002. In 2006, he received the Leonard Tow Humanism in Medicine Award. Dr Grubb lives with his wife Barbara and his children Helen and Alex. For relaxation, he writes and publishes prose and poetry and collects fountain pens.

CHAPTER 1

Introduction

The Fainting Phenomenon is intended to help the large numbers of people whose lives are negatively affected by the threat—and the reality—of fainting. Research has discovered a lot about what causes fainting. However, we have a long way to go, especially in educating both physicians and the public.

We now know that the brain and the autonomic nervous system (ANS) automatically regulate many of the normal functions of the body. This is especially true when the functions are outside of your conscious control, such as control of your heart rate, blood pressure, body temperature, and bowel function.

Think of your brain as being like a thermostat. The thermostat in your home automatically instructs your heating system to turn on and off in response to changes in temperature. Once you set the thermostat, you do not usually have to think about it after that. But what if your furnace suddenly was not putting out the heat needed to keep you warm? You might assume that something is wrong with the furnace—all you know is that you are cold. What if, when you called in a repair person, you were told that there was nothing wrong with your furnace? Hopefully, the repair person would next think to check your thermostat to see if it was working properly. But think how you would feel if, instead of checking the thermostat, the repair person concluded that your blue-tinged skin and goose bumps "must all be in your imagination."

This is what can happen to someone with a disorder that causes fainting. Your brain and nervous system work in much the same way as the thermostat. You are not normally aware of your brain and ANS functioning, only of the end results . . . or lack of them. Imagine a situation in which you went to your doctor and reported that your heart seemed to stop at times. It would be both upsetting and frustrating if, after checking your heart, your doctor concluded that since there was nothing wrong with the heart itself, the problem must be "in your head." In a way, the doctor might be right, but not the way you think.

The stopping of your heart might actually be due to some malfunction of the signals sent to the heart from the brain and the ANS. The furnace—your heart—might check out okay, but still not be working properly because of problems with the thermostat—your brain—or the wiring connecting the two—the ANS. A whole new branch of medicine has developed to look at symptoms caused by malfunctioning of your brain and/or ANS.

It is interesting to note that a number of people with disorders of the ANS have been misdiagnosed as having other disorders. For example, people with some types of ANS disorders can experience extreme fatigue because of the way the brain and ANS regulate blood pressure and heart rate. These individuals may be mistakenly diagnosed as having chronic fatigue syndrome. It is estimated that as many as 20% of the people diagnosed as having chronic fatigue syndrome may actually have ANS problems. Why is this important? There is currently no uniformly effective treatment for chronic fatigue syndrome. ANS disorders, on the other hand, can often be successfully treated, allowing the person to return to normal functioning. When the correct diagnosis is missed, it can be tragic for individuals who may continue to be almost totally incapacitated; they may not be able to function. The symptoms can have negative effects on all aspects of their life, including personal relationships, the ability to hold a job, and enjoyment of hobbies, among others.

Knowledge is power! It is important for you to know that symptoms such as fainting or chronic fatigue may possibly be a sign of a disorder of your ANS. Just because the underlying cause for these symptoms does not show up in a basic physical examination or a blood test is not proof that your problems are psychosomatic, that is, caused by psychological instead of physical problems.

CHAPTER 2

The fainting phenomenon

This book is all about fainting—losing consciousness and, unless something or someone prevents it, slumping to the floor. A faint usually does not last very long, and you typically regain consciousness within a few seconds or minutes, even when nothing is done to awaken you. (The medical term for fainting, which appears throughout this book, is syncope.) As you continue to read, you will see that there is a very broad range of underlying causes for syncope—the fainting phenomenon. Some of the causes are not too serious in themselves, while others can be lethal.

Fainting is no minor matter

Fainting is more common than you might think. It is estimated that about one-third of all adults will experience at least one fainting episode at some time in their life. People who experience recurring fainting episodes can have a reduced quality of life, comparable to that resulting from such debilitating conditions as severe rheumatoid arthritis or low back pain. And, as you might imagine, the more frequent the fainting episodes, the greater the impact on quality of life. One example of a negative effect on the quality of life is that the threat of fainting may bar someone from safely driving a car or other vehicle.

Do not write off fainting as a minor inconvenience—it can pose a real health risk. It is estimated that fainting accounts for 3% of all visits to the emergency room and up to 6% of all hospital admissions. People who faint without warning can be hurt when they fall. These falls can cause serious injuries such as a subdural hematoma (a leakage of blood in the brain) or fractures of the bones in the face, skull, arms, and legs. In older individuals, a single fainting episode can cause injuries serious enough to require permanent placement in a nursing home. As American humorist Will Rogers once commented, "it's not the fall that hurts, it's that sudden stop at the end." And recurring fainting episodes are sometimes the only symptom that precedes sudden death.

What causes most faints?

Fainting is a symptom, rather than a disease or condition. You typically faint when there is a decrease in the amount of oxygen-carrying blood flowing to your brain. So, fainting is actually caused by a short-term reduction in blood pressure to your brain—a type of temporary low blood pressure (hypotension). A decrease in blood flow as brief as 8–10 seconds may cause you to faint. When the cells of your brain are not able to get enough oxygen from your blood to function properly, you lose consciousness.

Sometimes you may first feel dizzy or light-headed—it's a warning to you that you are about to faint. Fainting often occurs when you sit up from a lying position or stand up from a lying or sitting position. An inability to move to an upright position without developing symptoms is called orthostatic (having to do with your position) intolerance. Orthostatic (postural) hypotension is the term used to describe a drop in blood pressure that occurs when your position or posture becomes upright.

If you fall when you faint, your blood pressure usually comes back up to more normal levels once you are on the ground, allowing you to regain consciousness. The rise in blood pressure may be due to your lying down, or sometimes the original cause of your fainting episode has passed. Keep in mind that trying to get up too quickly may lead to your fainting again.

Under certain circumstances, even normal people may develop the symptoms that often precede a faint or even experience the faint itself. This would typically be caused by a combination of circumstances. Let us say that you are in a warm environment, which would cause the blood vessels carrying blood to your skin to become larger. Next, you hyperventilate—breathing more rapidly than normal. This results in the blood vessels in your brain contracting, or becoming smaller. If you now suddenly stand up from a crouched position, blood will pool in your lower body and have a difficult battle against gravity to flow back up to your brain. The result: you get symptoms or you actually lose consciousness.

Your blood pressure can also drop when you lose a lot of the fluid from your system, decreasing the amount of blood available to reach the brain. This can result from dehydration due to excessive sweating or urination or from fluid losses during diarrhea. Of course, your blood volume also drops if your lose blood due to an injury.

There are a number of factors that can lower your blood pressure and decrease the supply of oxygen to your brain. In this book, we will deal in some detail with the most common causes underlying the fainting phenomenon in people who go to a doctor for this problem.

Looking forward...

To make it easier to understand what can go wrong in blood pressure control, we will first look at how your body normally controls blood pressure. Chapter 3 contains some useful information on those aspects of the nervous system most involved in controlling and maintaining blood pressure.

The normal nervous system

It is not the purpose of this chapter to give a complete and detailed description of the human nervous system. It would require an entire book—a large one—to do this effectively. However, there are certain functions of the nervous system that have a direct effect on how your body automatically controls your blood pressure.

Introduction to your nervous system

Your nervous system has three main functions: the sensory (afferent) function, the integration function, and the motor (efferent) function (see Figure 3-1).

• *Sensory function:* In its sensory function, your nervous system senses changes inside and outside your body. This is your nervous system's information-gathering phase. For example, seeing an angry bear in your path causes your sensory nerves to send certain messages. Different messages are sent if your sensory nerves are stimulated by a change in your internal temperature, such as when you are running a fever.

• *Integration function:* The term *integration* basically means bringing parts of something together. Therefore, the integration function refers to the nervous system analyzing the information gained in its sensory function so that something can be done about it. Some of this information is stored for future use. Your integration function also makes decisions about appropriate behavior in response to this information, that is, it translates the incoming information into action. Go back to the angry bear for a minute. The integration function of your nervous system processes the information that there is a dangerous animal ahead and decides to initiate certain physical reactions to help avoid that danger. That is where the motor function comes in.

• *Motor function:* You usually think of a motor as doing something. So, it will come as no surprise that your nervous system's motor function refers to the behavior—the action—that results from the information gained in its sensory function and analyzed in its integration function. In its motor function, the nervous system responds to stimuli by initiating action. These actions typically include contracting your muscles or causing your glands to produce and release substances such as hormones. You have probably heard of the "fight or flight" response. When you are in danger, your body responds in ways that allows you to face the threat: fight—or escape, take flight.

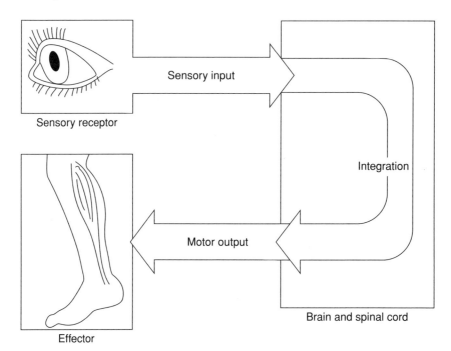

Figure 3-1 Three main functions of the nervous system: the sensory (afferent) function, the integration function, and the motor (efferent) function.

Did you know?

The fight or flight response is a combination of physical responses to danger, either real or imagined. Here is what happens: The pupils of your eyes dilate or grow larger. Your heart begins to beat more quickly and strongly, and your blood pressure rises. Blood vessels carrying blood to organs that are not needed to either fight or run away constrict, that is, become smaller. This allows processes not necessary at that moment, such as digesting food, to be temporarily put on hold. At the same time, vessels carrying blood to the organs involved in fighting danger—skeletal muscles, heart muscles, brain, and lungs—become larger, resulting in a greater blood supply. Small air tubes in your lungs become larger so that more oxygen can get into your blood. Your body converts stored carbohydrate (glycogen) to blood sugar for extra energy. And, your adrenal glands produce substances that make all of these effects more intense and long lasting. All in all, the body goes through a complex series of changes to enable you to either fight or to run away to fight again some other day.

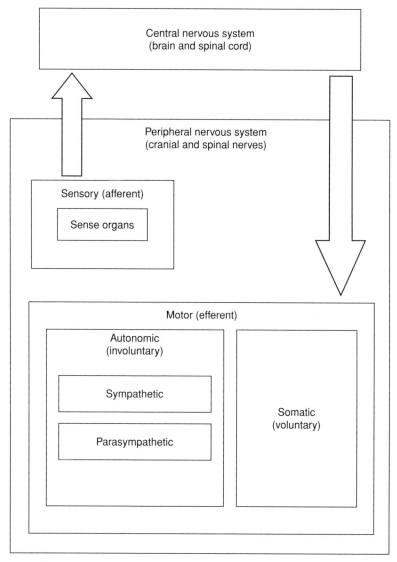

Figure 3-2 Two main parts of the nervous system: the central nervous system and the peripheral nervous system.

Your nervous system has two main parts: your central nervous system (CNS) and your peripheral nervous system (PNS) (see Figure 3-2).

Your central nervous system

Your CNS consists of your brain and spinal cord. The brain is the driving force for almost all of the functions of your nervous system.

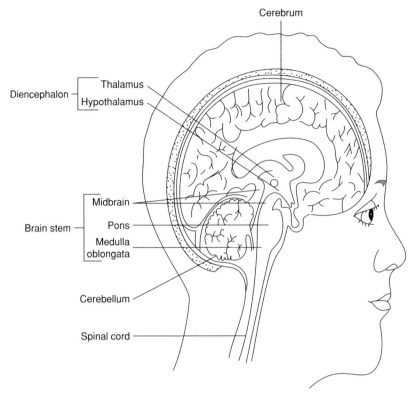

Cerebrum

Diencephalon
Thalamus
Hypothalamus

Brain stem
Midbrain
Pons
Medulla oblongata

Cerebellum

Spinal cord

Figure 3-3 Four main parts of the human brain: the brainstem, the diencephalon, the cerebrum, and the cerebellum.

The human brain is a mushroom-shaped organ that has four principal parts (see Figure 3-3):
• *Brainstem:* Your brainstem is actually a continuation of your spinal cord. Keeping the mushroom example in mind, you might think of the brainstem as the stalk of the mushroom. The brainstem consists of the medulla oblongata, pons, and midbrain.
• *Diencephalon:* The area above the brainstem is called the diencephalon. It consists mainly of two glands: the thalamus and the hypothalamus. In spite of its small size, the hypothalamus is known as the body's "master gland" because it controls so many activities in the body, a number of which are involved in maintaining homeostasis. For example, the hypothalamus controls and organizes the activities of the autonomic nervous system (ANS) and regulates the release of many hormones from the pituitary gland.
• *Cerebrum:* The cerebrum is the part of the brain that spreads over the diencephalon, filling much of the cranium (skull). It has two sides called hemispheres.
• *Cerebellum:* The cerebellum is the part of the brain located below the cerebrum and behind the brainstem.

In order for your brain to carry out its many essential functions, it needs a very good oxygen supply. A special set of blood vessels—your cerebrovascular (cerebro = brain; vascular = blood vessels) system—is responsible for carrying oxygen and nutrients to all parts of your brain.

The principal nutrient that blood supplies to the brain is glucose, a type of simple sugar, which you may have heard being called blood sugar. Glucose is the primary energy source (fuel) for the brain. If the blood entering your brain contains too little glucose (hypoglycemia), you could experience symptoms such as dizziness, confusion, convulsions, and/or a loss of consciousness.

Cutting off the supply of oxygen-carrying blood to the brain—even for a very short period of time—will also cause unconsciousness. Brain cells must have oxygen in order to function. Without it, they stop carrying out the tremendous number of jobs they do in the body. Depriving the brain of oxygen for as little as 4 minutes may cause permanent injury to the brain.

Did you know...?

Although the brain accounts for only about 2% of your body's total weight, it needs about 20% of the oxygen used by your body.

Of course, your blood also carries other substances to your brain. Some of them are able to cross over the separating membrane and enter the cells of your brain; others are not able to pass out of the blood and into the brain. The "blood–brain barrier" refers to the mechanism by which the walls of the tiny blood vessels—capillaries—in the brain allow only small molecules and larger molecules of certain substances to pass into your brain cells. You will sometimes hear this term used to describe the activity of a drug that either can or cannot cross the blood–brain barrier.

Your spinal cord runs down from the brainstem and through a canal in your spinal column, your backbone. By passing through the spinal canal, your spinal cord is essentially protected by a ring of bone. Your spine has 31 separate segments, each of which is the source of one pair of spinal nerves. The 31 pairs of spinal nerves are named and numbered according to the level at which they emerge along the spinal cord. You have

- 8 pairs of cervical nerves in the neck region,
- 12 pairs of thoracic nerves in the chest region,
- 5 pairs of lumbar nerves in the lower back,
- 5 pairs of sacral nerves in the pelvic region, and
- 1 pair of coccygeal nerves at the very bottom of your spinal column—your "tailbone."

Your peripheral nervous system

The PNS consists of the nerves that arise from the brain (cranial nerves) and spinal cord (spinal nerves). The nerves in the PNS carry nerve impulses both into and out of the CNS. (Nerve impulses are like tiny electric currents being carried along nerve cells.)

Some nerve cells, or neurons, connect the CNS to sensory receptors. These sensory (afferent) neurons carry impulses from the sensory receptors to the CNS—they handle incoming information. Sensory receptors do the actual "sensing" of changes inside and outside the body, as was mentioned earlier. Some sensory receptors respond to touch, while others respond to pressure, cold, light, heat, sound, and other stimuli. At the receptor, the sensed stimulus is converted into a nerve impulse.

Neurons that start in the CNS and carry nerve impulses to the muscles and glands that are targeted by the motor functions of the nervous system are called motor (efferent) neurons—they handle outgoing orders. A third type of neuron is called an association neuron (or interneuron). Association neurons, which are found in the CNS, act as bridges, carrying nerve impulses from sensory to motor neurons.

Your PNS is further divided into two parts: the somatic nervous system and the ANS.

Your somatic nervous system

You are probably more aware of your somatic nervous system than of your ANS. Its sensory neurons pick up information from special receptors in your head, trunk, arms, and legs and send it to the CNS. The motor neurons of the somatic nervous system carry nerve impulses only to your skeletal muscles. These nerve impulses cause muscles, which are attached to bones, to contract, resulting in movement of the bones at a joint. Think about what happens when you bend your arm at the elbow. You are aware of accomplishing this movement by contracting your biceps muscle (located at the front of your arm, between your shoulder and elbow). However, the actual contraction is the result of nerve impulses carried to the muscle by way of the somatic nervous system's motor neurons.

Your autonomic nervous system

When you discuss the subject of fainting, you are most interested in the part of the nervous system called the ANS. The first part of the word *autonomic* should give you a hint about its function. This is your involuntary, or "automatic," nervous system. It is involved in the body functions that occur without you having to think about them. For example, the ANS regulates the smooth muscle found in the walls of your organs, cardiac (heart) muscle, and your glands— usually without your even being aware of it. The ANS consists mostly of motor neurons, which carry nerve impulses from the CNS to these different types of muscles and glands.

The ANS has two branches: the sympathetic division and the parasympathetic division. For the most part, both of these divisions send nerve impulses to your muscles and glands.

Your body typically tries to maintain a state called homeostasis. This means automatically adjusting different processes within the body to maintain a relatively constant balance (within a certain range). Body temperature is a good example. No matter what the outside temperature is, your body automatically makes adjustments to try to maintain 98.6°F, or whatever is a normal body temperature for you. In order to maintain homeostasis, the two divisions of the ANS often have opposite effects, enabling them to maintain the proper balance.

As a rule, sympathetic neurons promote activities and processes that use energy. Parasympathetic neurons, on the other hand, tend to have effects that save and restore energy in your body. Take the activities of your heart—your sympathetic nervous system speeds up the rate at which your heart beats, while your parasympathetic nervous system slows it down.

The main function of the sympathetic division is to counteract the effects of the parasympathetic division just enough to carry out the processes in the body that require energy. However, when you are under extreme stress—fight or flight—the sympathetic division becomes dominant.

Table 3-1 shows just a few of the activities of the sympathetic and parasympathetic divisions of the ANS. (Remember that "secretion" refers to the production and release of something, such as an enzyme or hormone, from a gland or tissue.)

Nerve pathways in the ANS consist of two motor neurons. One goes from the CNS to a ganglion, which is a small knot or group of nerve cells. The second neuron stretches from the ganglion to the muscle or gland where the nerve impulse causes a response. Think of a nerve impulse as having a journey that is in two stages. It first travels from the CNS to the ganglion and then continues to its final destination—a muscle or gland. The first neuron is called a preganglionic neuron, which simply means that it is located between the brain or spinal cord and the ganglion. If you are catching on to how scientists name things, you may already have figured out that the neuron between the ganglion and the muscle or gland is called a postganglionic neuron.

Table 3-1 Some activities of the sympathetic and parasympathetic divisions of the ANS.

Glands/muscles/ responses affected	Sympathetic stimulation	Parasympathetic stimulation
Heart muscle	Increases heart rate and strength of contraction	Decreases heart rate and strength of contraction
Blood vessels	Constricts blood vessel walls (vasoconstriction)	No known effect
Kidney	Stimulates secretion of renin (an enzyme that helps raise blood pressure); decreases urine volume	No known effect
Salivary (saliva-producing) glands	Decreases secretion of saliva	Stimulates secretion of saliva
Tear glands	No known effect	Stimulates secretion of tears

Neurons: basic nerve cells

Throughout the previous discussion, you have come across the term *neuron*, which is just another name for a nerve cell. Neurons carry nerve impulses for thinking, controlling muscle activity, and regulating glands, among countless other functions.

Neurons have three parts: the cell body, an axon, and dendrites (see Figure 3-4). Most neurons have several main dendrites extending from the cell body. The dendrites are usually short, thick, and highly branched. A dendrite receives incoming nerve impulses from either a sensory receptor or another nerve cell and then transmits them to the cell body. Each neuron has only one axon, which is a long, thin extension of the cell body. The axon receives nerve impulses from the cell body and sends them to another neuron or to a tissue.

How is the nerve impulse transmitted from one neuron to another? The dendrites of one neuron do not actually touch the axon of the next neuron in

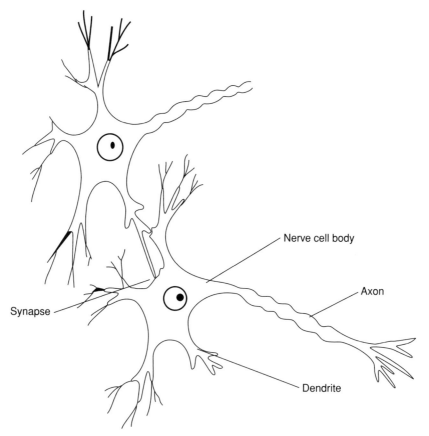

Figure 3-4 Three parts of a neuron: the cell body, the axon, and the dendrites. A synapse is a tiny space between the axon of one neuron and the dendrites of the next one.

line. And, a nerve impulse cannot just jump over the tiny space—synapse—between the axon of one neuron and the dendrites of the next one. Next we will see what happens actually.

The end of the axon has many fine threadlike structures called axon terminals. The axon terminals, in turn, have bulblike structures (synaptic end bulbs) containing sacs (synaptic vesicles) that store chemical substances called neurotransmitters. When a neurotransmitter is released by the axon, it travels over the synapse and "docks" at a receptor on a dendrite of the next neuron in line. Receptors typically are specific for a particular substance or family of substances. Therefore, dendrites must have different types of receptors. Which neurotransmitters are present determine whether a nerve impulse passes from one neuron to another or from a neuron to a tissue.

There is also a tiny space separating the axon of a postganglionic neuron and the muscle or gland to which it carries nerve impulses. A neuromuscular junction is the space between a neuron and a muscle cell; a neuroglandular junction separates a neuron from the gland it stimulates.

Did you know...?

A stimulus is a "stress" or change inside or outside the body that excites a nerve or muscle fiber. In any discussion of the nervous system, a stimulus typically refers to anything in the internal or external environment that can cause a neuron that is not carrying a nerve impulse to change its electrical charge so that it is able to carry the impulse. A nerve's degree of "excitability" is its ability to respond to a stimulus and to convert it into a nerve impulse.

Neurotransmitters can transmit one of the two types of messages. An excitatory transmission creates a new nerve impulse, causing the original impulse to continue. An inhibitory transmission, on the other hand, prevents the nerve impulse from continuing-basically, stopping the impulse in its tracks.

Did you know...?

A neuron can carry nerve impulses only one way. Therefore, nerve pathways always go from dendrites → the cell body → the axon → across the synapse by way of neurotransmitters → receptor cells on the dendrites of the next neuron or to the receptor cells of a muscle or gland.

A single neuron can receive both excitatory and inhibitory transmissions from many presynaptic neurons. It is then the job of the postsynaptic neuron to receive these signals, integrate them, and respond to the one that dominates. It is the balance between these opposite messages that determines the final effect on the postsynaptic neuron.

Table 3-2 Some common neurotransmitters and their functions.

Neurotransmitter	Location and function
Acetylcholine	Found in cerebral cortex of the brain, skeletal neuromuscular junctions, and the ANS. Usually excitatory.
Dopamine	Concentrated in the brain. Generally excitatory. Involved in emotional responses and subconscious movements of skeletal muscles. Decreased levels are associated with Parkinson's disease.
Epinephrine* (adrenaline)	Found in the CNS. Usually excitatory. Produces actions similar to those resulting from stimulation from the sympathetic division of the ANS. Increases blood pressure by increasing heart rate and constricting blood vessels. Predominantly released in response to low blood sugar (hypoglycemia), stress, and other stimuli. More potent than norepinephrine.
Norepinephrine* (noradrenaline)	Concentrated in brainstem and also found in other parts of the CNS. Released at some neuromuscular and neuroglandular junctions. Usually excitatory. Primarily released in response to low blood pressure (hypotension) and stress. Potent constrictor of blood vessels. May be related to arousal, dreaming, and mood regulation.
Serotonin	Found in the CNS. Generally inhibitory. May be involved in inducing sleep, sensory perception, temperature regulation, and mood control.

*Epinephrine and norepinephrine are two hormonal neurotransmitters that are grouped under the general heading of catecholamines.

Neurotransmitters

Neurotransmitters are made by the neuron out of amino acids, the building blocks of protein. There are an estimated 60 substances in the body that are thought to be neurotransmitters. The activities of the nervous system depend on proper levels and regulation of these neurotransmitters. Table 3-2 introduces you to a few common neurotransmitters, some of which may be familiar.

Looking forward...

Now you have a general idea of how your nervous system works. Chapter 4 provides an overview of the cardiovascular (cardio = heart; vascular = blood vessels) system and the normal regulation of blood pressure.

Reference

Tortora GJ. *Introduction to the Human Body: The Essentials of Anatomy and Physiology*, 4th edition. Menlo Park, CA: Biological Sciences Textbooks, Inc., 1997.

The normal cardiovascular system

In this chapter, you will learn how your cardiovascular system works. (As you saw in the last chapter, the term cardiovascular refers to your heart and blood vessels.) Your cardiovascular system, often under the direction of your autonomic nervous system (ANS) (see Chapter 3), is responsible for the control of blood pressure. This brief review of the normal cardiovascular system will make it easier to understand how abnormalities in this system (and in the ANS) can lead to too little oxygen-containing blood reaching the cells of the brain—the major cause of fainting.

Basics of the cardiovascular system

Your cardiovascular system consists of your heart and a network of several different types of blood vessels. As you will soon learn, your cardiovascular system is quite remarkable!

Did you know?

Even when you are at rest, your heart pumps more than 2000 gallons of blood in 24 hours? And, if all your blood vessels were laid out end to end, they would stretch an estimated 60,000 miles.

Together, the heart and blood vessels form two separate circulatory systems (see Figure 4-1).
• Pulmonary circulation carries blood to and from your heart to your lungs.
• Systemic circulation transports blood to and from your heart to all the other parts of your body.
You may sometimes see a mention of cerebral or hepatic circulation. Cerebral circulation refers to the circulation of blood in your brain—your cerebrovascular system. Hepatic circulation means blood circulation in your liver. However, both cerebral and hepatic circulation are actually part of systemic circulation.

Workings of your heart
Although it is only about the size of a closed fist, your heart plays an essential role in maintaining life. Your heart is located in your chest between your lungs. It is shaped somewhat like a cone. The larger part of the cone (base) is at the top and the blunted point (apex) is at the lower end, resting on your

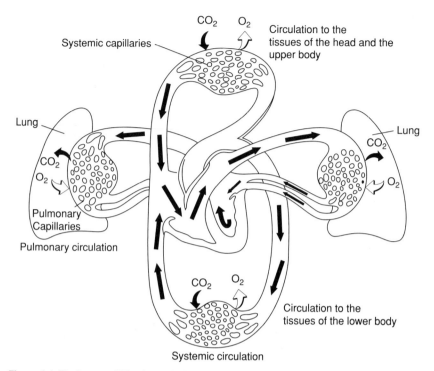

CO$_2$ O$_2$

Circulation to the tissues of the head and the upper body

Systemic capillaries

Lung

Lung

CO$_2$

CO$_2$

O$_2$

O$_2$

Pulmonary Capillaries

Pulmonary circulation

CO$_2$ O$_2$

Circulation to the tissues of the lower body

Systemic circulation

Figure 4-1 The heart and blood vessels form two separate circulatory systems: the pulmonary circulation and the systemic circulation.

diaphragm (a dome-shaped muscle stretching across the inside of your body and separating your chest from your abdomen) (see Figure 4-2).

The wall of your heart has three layers: the endocardium, the myocardium, and the epicardium.

• *Endocardium:* The endocardium lines the inside of the heart, covering the heart valves. It forms a continuous layer with the inner lining of the blood vessels carrying blood to and away from the heart.

• *Myocardium:* The myocardium consists of thick bundles of special cardiac muscle that do not occur anywhere else in the body. This cardiac muscle is designed for one function—to allow the heart to pump blood. Cardiac muscle is a type of involuntary muscle, meaning that it functions without you being aware of it.

• *Epicardium:* The epicardium is the thin outer layer of the heart wall.

Your heart actually functions as two separate pumps, both doing different but similar jobs at the same time. It has four chambers (see Figure 4-3). The two smaller, thinner-walled chambers (atria) at the top of the heart receive blood. The two larger chambers beneath the atria—the ventricles—are more muscular because their job is to act as pumping chambers. The right atrium and ventricle form the pump for pulmonary circulation, and the left atrium

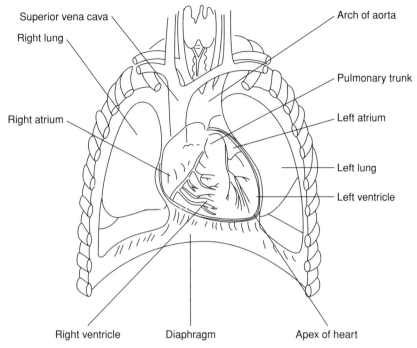

Superior vena cava

Right lung

Right atrium

Arch of aorta

Pulmonary trunk

Left atrium

Left lung

Left ventricle

Right ventricle   Diaphragm   Apex of heart

Figure 4-2 The heart is located between the lungs.

and ventricle pump blood throughout your systemic circulation. Therefore, the left ventricle has the thickest layer of cardiac muscle in its myocardium because it is responsible for pumping blood to a much larger area.

Did you know?

Although some of the terms used to describe the parts of the heart and blood vessels look pretty technical, they may be easier to understand than you think. Look at the parts that make up the word—they often give you a hint of its meaning. For example, *interatrial* describes something between the two atria and *interventricular* means between the two ventricles. Later in this discussion, you will see the word atrioventricular. Looking at the parts of the word, you may have already figured out that it refers to an atrium and a ventricle. Typically, this word is used to describe something located between an atrium and the ventricle below it.

A wall, called a septum, divides the left and right sides of the heart. (You may be familiar with the term "deviated septum," which refers to a bend, or deviation, in the wall-like structure that divides the two sides of your nose.)

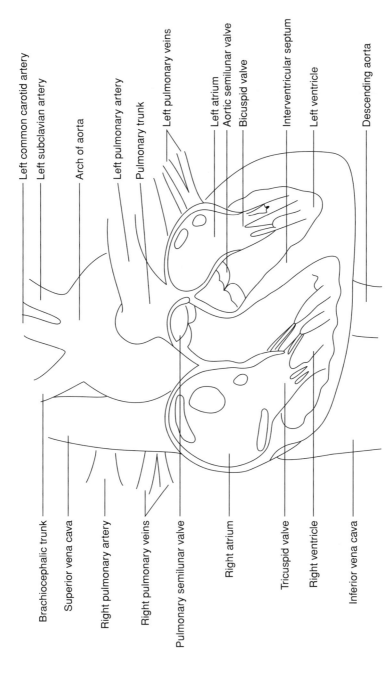

Left common carotid artery

Left subclavian artery

Arch of aorta

Left pulmonary artery

Pulmonary trunk

Left pulmonary veins

Left atrium

Aortic semilunar valve

Bicuspid valve

Interventricular septum

Left ventricle

Descending aorta

Brachiocephalic trunk

Superior vena cava

Right pulmonary artery

Right pulmonary veins

Pulmonary semilunar valve

Right atrium

Tricuspid valve

Right ventricle

Inferior vena cava

Figure 4-3 Four chambers of the heart: right atrium, right ventricle, left atrium, and left ventricle.

The portion of the septum that is located between the two atria is called the interatrial septum, and the interventricular septum separates the two ventricles.

The heart has a system of valves to keep blood moving in the right direction. These valves are flaps of dense connective tissue that open to let blood pass through and then close to prevent blood from flowing backward. There are two atrioventricular (AV) valves. As the name suggests, each of these valves is located between an atrium and the ventricle beneath it. The AV valve between the right atrium and ventricle is called the tricuspid valve. A cusp is a flap, and the tricuspid valve consists of three flaps that allow blood to flow from the right atrium into the right ventricle. The AV valve on the left side of the heart is called the bicuspid, or mitral, valve.

The other two heart valves are called semilunar valves because they are shaped somewhat like a half moon. These valves prevent blood that is being pumped out of the heart and into the arteries from flowing backward into the ventricles.

A look at your blood vessels

Blood pumped out of your heart is carried to every cell in your body by a remarkable system of blood vessels. Think of arteries as carrying blood away from the heart and veins as returning blood back to the heart. The larger arteries leading away from the heart branch into medium-sized arteries and then into very small arteries, called arterioles. The arterioles further divide to form capillaries, which are extremely tiny, microscopic, vessels located in the tissues of the body. The thin walls of the capillaries allow oxygen and nutrients to pass out of blood and into the body's cells. At the same time, blood in the capillaries absorbs carbon dioxide and other waste products to be excreted (eliminated) from the body. The capillaries then join together to form venules (tiny veins), which rejoin further to form larger veins that ultimately go back to the heart. As you can see, this system of blood vessels forms a circuit through which blood continually circulates.

Although arteries and veins both have three layers, their structures are somewhat different. As you can see in Figure 4-4, the inner layer, or endothelium, of arteries and veins is called the tunica intima, which literally means inside coat. The middle layer, or tunica media, consists of smooth muscle and elastic tissue. The outer layer is called the tunica externa or the external coat.

The layer of smooth muscle and elastic fibers—the tunica media—is much thicker in arteries than in veins. Why do arteries need all that muscle and elasticity? These vessels have to be strong to withstand the force of blood being pumped out of the heart. Arteries also need to be elastic so that they can grow larger (dilate or expand) and become smaller (constrict or contract). Arteries expand when blood is forced out of the heart as its ventricles contract, and they contract to help force blood through the circulatory system.

Another important difference is that the inner layer, or tunica intima, of a vein folds over to form valves. Why are the valves in your veins important? Think about blood flow to your legs, for instance. Blood is pumped down through

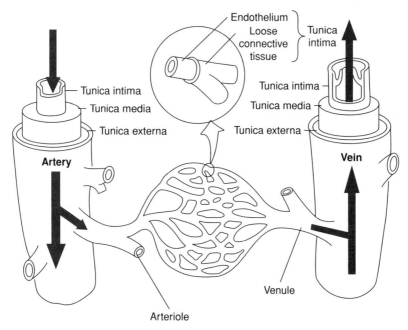

Figure 4-4 Components of the arteries and the veins.

the arteries and arterioles in your legs. Each time a blood vessel divides to form many smaller vessels, the pressure pushing the blood forward becomes less. By the time blood reaches your capillaries, there is very little pressure behind it. However, after leaving your capillaries, your blood now has to move upward—against gravity—to get back to your heart. Therefore, as blood is slowly pushed upward, the valves in your veins open to allow it to move toward the heart and then close to prevent the blood from being pulled backward into your legs.

Your two circulatory systems

The easiest way to understand your two circulatory systems is to follow some blood as it travels throughout your body. Your blood starts its journey after it has given up its oxygen and nutrients to the cells of your body. This "tired blood" enters the right atrium of the heart through two large veins, called the superior and the inferior vena cava. The blood passes from the right atrium into the right ventricle, where, as the heart contracts, it is pumped out into the pulmonary trunk. The pulmonary trunk quickly divides into the right and left pulmonary arteries, each of which goes to one of your lungs. The blood flows into smaller vessels in your lungs, where it picks up oxygen and gets rid of carbon dioxide. The newly oxygenated blood travels through four pulmonary veins back to your heart's left atrium. This cycle from the heart to the lungs and back to the heart again is your pulmonary circulation.

In your systemic circulation, the oxygenated blood that has been returned to the left atrium passes into the left ventricle and is pumped out into a large artery called the ascending aorta, which, as the name suggests, is located above the heart. From the ascending aorta, oxygen-rich blood passes into the

- coronary arteries or arteries in the heart muscle itself,
- arch of the aorta, which branches off into the carotid arteries going up to the brain through the neck,
- thoracic aorta, which is the large artery in the chest area, and
- abdominal aorta, which is the large artery in the abdomen.

Further branching of these major arteries into smaller arteries allows blood to travel to all the parts of your body. The blood follows a path through smaller arteries, arterioles, capillaries, venules, and veins mentioned earlier before being returned to the right atrium of your heart.

Did you know?

We typically think of arteries as carrying oxygen-rich blood, and veins as carrying oxygen-poor blood. This is true in the case of systemic circulation in which arteries carry oxygen-rich blood away from the heart and veins return oxygen-poor blood to it. However, the reverse is true in pulmonary circulation—pulmonary arteries carry oxygen-poor blood from your heart to your lungs and pulmonary veins return oxygen-rich blood to your heart.

About your heartbeat

A single heartbeat takes less than a second. The period from the beginning of one heartbeat to the beginning of the next is called the cardiac cycle. The cardiac cycle has two basic phases: systole and diastole.

Systole refers to the contraction of the chambers in the heart, especially the ventricles. Here is what happens during systole. As pressure builds up in the ventricle, first the bicuspid and tricuspid valves close to prevent backflow of blood into the atria. Then the semilunar valves open to allow blood to be pumped out of—or ejected from—the heart. The ventricles contract, ejecting blood into the pulmonary artery (on the right) and the aorta (on the left) and then relax.

The relaxation phase is called diastole. The semilunar valves close at the beginning of diastole to prevent blood from backing up into the relaxed ventricles. At the same time the bicuspid and tricuspid valves open to allow blood to start draining into the ventricles from the atria. Actually, about 75% of the blood in each atrium drains into the ventricle before the atrium contracts, forcing the remaining 25% of blood downward. When the diastolic phase is almost over, the atria contract to send the remaining blood into the ventricles. Then it is time for systole again.

Here are a few more terms that will be useful later. Cardiac output typically refers to the amount of blood your left ventricle ejects into the aorta during systole in a minute's time. (Depending on the definition you use, it can also be a measure of the amount of blood ejected by your right ventricle.) Cardiac output is calculated by multiplying the amount of blood ejected during one contraction—the stroke volume—by the number of heartbeats per minute. For example, an adult at rest might have a stroke volume of about 2.4 fluid ounces (70 ml) and a heart rate of about 75 beats per minute. Multiplying 2.4 fluid ounces by 75 gives you a cardiac output of about 180 fluid ounces (or 1.4 gallons) of blood ejected per minute.

What makes your heart beat?

Your heart has its own electrical, or conduction, system that regulates your heartbeat. Your heart's conduction system consists of special tissue found nowhere else in the body. This tissue can best be described as a cross between muscle and nervous tissue. The five main parts of your heart's electrical system, as illustrated in Figure 4-5, are
- sinoatrial (SA) node,
- AV node,
- AV bundle or bundle of His,
- bundle branches, and
- Purkinje fibers.

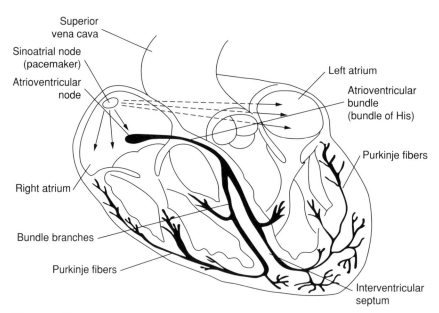

Figure 4-5 Five main parts of the heart's electrical system: the sinoatrial node, the atrioventricular node, the atrioventricular bundle or bundle of His, the bundle branches, and the Purkinje fibers.

Heart muscle is unique among the muscles in the body because it does not require stimulation from the central nervous system (CNS) in order to contract. The SA node (or sinus node), which is located in the wall of the right atrium, is called the pacemaker because it initiates each heartbeat and sets the pace for the heart. The SA node generates nerve impulses faster than the other, slower parts of the heart's electrical system. An impulse that begins in the SA node quickly spreads out over both atria, causing them to contract simultaneously.

The impulse next travels to the AV node, which is located in the interatrial septum—the wall separating the two atria. The AV node slows down the nerve impulse, which allows the atria enough time to finish contracting and emptying blood into the ventricles before the larger chambers begin to contract.

The nerve impulse then goes from the AV node to special conducting fibers— the AV bundle—located at the top of the interventricular septum. The impulse finally travels from the AV bundle through the right and left bundle branches located in the interventricular septum. Both ventricles actually contract when their myocardium is stimulated by impulses from tiny muscle fibers, called Purkinje fibers, which emerge from the bundle branches and spread throughout the muscle of the ventricle walls.

ANS and your heart

Although heart muscle does not rely on your nervous system to contract, the ANS does play an important role in controlling the rate of your heartbeat. Specialized nerves in one division of the ANS act as "brakes" to slow down heart rate, while nerves in the other division act as "accelerators" to speed it up.

There is a particular group of neurons, or nerve cells, called the cardiovascular center, which is located in the medulla oblongata (see Chapter 3) of the brain. The cardiovascular center affects heart rate and regulates how hard the heart contracts. (As you will soon see, it also controls the diameter of blood vessels.) For example, stimulating a particular part of the cardiovascular center causes neurons in the sympathetic division of the peripheral nervous system (PNS) to activate special accelerator nerves in the conduction system of the atria and ventricles. The accelerator nerves cause an increase in heart rate and greater strength of contraction by releasing a hormone neurotransmitter called norepinephrine.

The cardiovascular center is also the source of parasympathetic fibers that reach the heart by way of the vagus nerves. If this part of your cardiovascular center is stimulated, nerve impulses are transmitted along the parasympathetic fibers to the conduction system and atria. These impulses cause the release of the neurotransmitter acetylcholine, which slows down the SA and AV nodes and decreases the rate of heartbeat and strength of the contractions. When your body is at rest, the parasympathetic division of the ANS controls the heart, and your heart rate is very slow. However, when you are active or under stress, the sympathetic division of the ANS stimulates the heart to contract more forcefully and to speed up your heart rate.

As you can see, the overall effect of the ANS on the heart is the result of opposite actions—stimulation from sympathetic fibers and inhibition from parasympathetic fibers. How does the cardiovascular center know whether to stimulate sympathetic or parasympathetic responses? As you will see later, receptors in the cardiovascular system report conditions, such as changes in blood pressure, to the brain so that a proper balance of stimulation and inhibition can be maintained.

ANS and your blood vessels

A special group of neurons located in the cardiovascular center is called the vasomotor center. The vasomotor center is part of the sympathetic division of the ANS. It is in charge of controlling the size of the hollow area inside a blood vessel, or lumen (see Figure 4-4), especially in the arterioles located in the skin and abdomen.

Under normal conditions, the walls of your arterioles are moderately constricted most of the time due to sympathetic impulses sent to the smooth muscles in the vessel walls. This process, called vasoconstriction, reduces the size of the lumen. A decrease in lumen size typically increases blood pressure. A decrease in these sympathetic impulses causes an enlargement of the lumen—vasodilation—and a resulting reduction in blood pressure. Therefore, the sympathetic division of the ANS is actually responsible for both vasoconstriction and vasodilation of your arterioles.

Did you know?

It is interesting to note that autonomic control of the heart is the result of opposing sympathetic and parasympathetic stimulation. Autonomic control of blood vessels, however, is exclusively the result of more or less sympathetic stimulation.

Looking at blood pressure

Any discussion of fainting has to center on blood pressure. Blood pressure is defined as the pressure that blood exerts on the inside wall of an artery. It is given as two measurements—systolic and diastolic blood pressures. The systolic reading measures the force of blood pressing outward on the artery wall during systole, when the heart is contracting. The diastolic reading measures the remaining force exerted against artery walls during diastole, when the heart muscle is relaxed. Blood pressure is measured in millimeters of mercury (mm Hg). As you might expect, systolic pressure is much higher than diastolic pressure. Table 4-1 shows the classifications for normal, high-normal, high, and low blood pressures.

Table 4-1 Blood pressure classifications.

Blood pressure	Systolic blood pressure (mm Hg)	Diastolic blood pressure (mm Hg)
Normal	Less than 130	Less than 85
High-normal	130–139	85–89
High blood pressure	140 or greater	90 or greater
Low blood pressure	90 or less	—

What determines blood pressure? There are three factors:

• *Cardiac output*, the amount of blood your ventricle ejects in a minute, is the main factor in determining blood pressure.

• *Blood volume* is the total amount of blood being circulated throughout your body at any one time, typically about 5 quarts. When your blood volume falls, such as during a hemorrhage (large loss of blood), your blood pressure also drops. If your blood volume increases, your blood pressure goes up. For example, a high intake of salt typically causes you to retain extra fluid in your body, increasing your blood volume and raising your blood pressure.

• *Peripheral resistance* refers to the opposition to the flow of blood that results from friction between blood and blood vessel walls. Larger blood vessels, such as arteries and veins, have lower peripheral resistance than smaller vessels, such as arterioles, venules, and capillaries. The ability of arterioles to change lumen size by constricting and expanding helps them control peripheral resistance and regulate blood pressure.

How blood pressure is regulated

For optimum health, blood pressure needs to be kept within a normal range. High blood pressure can do a great deal of damage to the heart, brain, and kidneys. Low blood pressure, on the other hand, can result in inadequate oxygen and nutrients being delivered to the cells of the body, including those of your brain. If blood pressure drops low enough, it can result in a loss of consciousness or fainting.

In order to maintain blood pressure within a normal range, the cardiovascular center in the brain receives input from a number of sources. These sources include baroreceptors, chemoreceptors, hormones, and higher brain centers.

Baroreceptors

Baroreceptors are receptors that are sensitive to blood pressure changes. These structures are located in the arch of the aorta, in an enlarged area of the neck arteries called the carotid sinus, and in the right atrium. An increase in blood pressure causes the baroreceptors to send nerve impulses to stimulate the part of the cardiovascular center that sends inhibitory impulses to the heart. This results in more parasympathetic impulses being sent along the vagus nerves to the heart.

The increase in parasympathetic activity reduces heart rate and the force of the contractions, thereby lowering the amount of blood ejected with each contraction and reducing blood pressure. At the same time, the vasomotor center also sends fewer of the sympathetic impulses to the nerves that cause blood vessels to constrict and raise blood pressure.

These two activities—increased parasympathetic activity in the heart and lower sympathetic impulses to the blood vessels—both help lower blood pressure.

What happens when your blood pressure falls? In this case, the baroreceptors stop stimulating the cardiovascular center in the brain. This results in an increase in heart rate and force of contraction, higher cardiac output, and a constriction of blood vessels, all of which help increase your blood pressure to normal levels. Figure 4-6 illustrates what happens when your blood pressure drops.

Chemoreceptors

Chemoreceptors are special neurons that are sensitive to chemical substances in the blood. Your chemoreceptors are located in two carotid bodies (small structures found in the neck arteries) and in aortic bodies (located in the arch of the aorta). Chemoreceptors respond to abnormally low levels of oxygen and higher than normal levels of carbon dioxide and hydrogen in the blood. When these conditions are present, the chemoreceptors send impulses to the vasomotor center, which then increases sympathetic stimulation of the arterioles, resulting in vasoconstriction and an increase in blood pressure.

Hormones

Hormones are substances produced by one tissue in the body and carried by the bloodstream to other tissues, where they alter the physiological activity. Enzymes are substances that affect the speed of a chemical change. Several hormones and enzymes are especially important in blood pressure control:

• *Epinephrine and norepinephrine*—Both epinephrine and norepinephrine, which are produced by the medulla oblongata of the brain, raise blood pressure by increasing heart rate and the force of heart contractions and by causing arterioles in the skin and abdomen to constrict.

• *Renin*—A decrease in blood pressure causes the kidneys to secrete an enzyme called renin. Renin raises blood pressure in two ways. It not only causes vasoconstriction, but it also increases blood volume by influencing your kidneys to retain fluid.

• *Atrial natriuretic peptide (ANP)*—A hormone called ANP lowers blood pressure by causing vasodilation and by decreasing blood volume through promoting water and salt loss in urine.

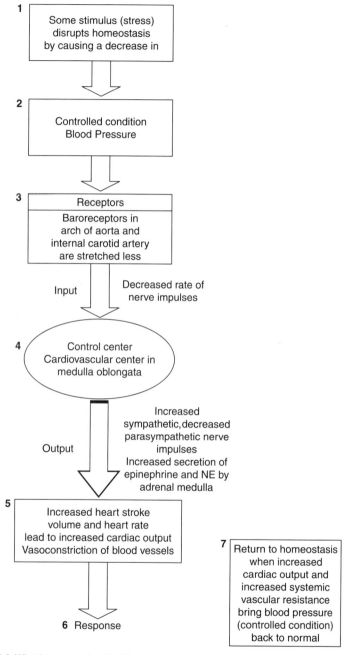

1 Some stimulus (stress) disrupts homeostasis by causing a decrease in

2 Controlled condition Blood Pressure

3 Receptors
Baroreceptors in arch of aorta and internal carotid artery are stretched less

Input   Decreased rate of nerve impulses

4 Control center
Cardiovascular center in medulla oblongata

Output

Increased sympathetic, decreased parasympathetic nerve impulses
Increased secretion of epinephrine and NE by adrenal medulla

5 Increased heart stroke volume and heart rate lead to increased cardiac output
Vasoconstriction of blood vessels

7 Return to homeostasis when increased cardiac output and increased systemic vascular resistance bring blood pressure (controlled condition) back to normal

6 Response

Figure 4-6 What happens when the blood pressure drops.

Did you know?

Did you ever wonder how alcohol lowers blood pressure? Follow along with the process. Alcohol inhibits the release of antidiuretic hormone (ADH). You may recognize the word diuretic in this term. Diuretics are sometimes called "water pills" because they cause you to excrete more urine. So, an antidiuretic would decrease urine loss. Therefore, inhibiting ADH results in fewer sympathetic impulses from the vasomotor center, ultimately leading to vasodilation, increased urination, and lower blood pressure. (You should be aware that chronic high use of alcohol may lead to hypertension.)

Higher brain centers

You probably know from personal experience that your blood pressure also responds to strong emotions. How does this happen? It depends on your higher brain center. Emotions such as intense anger cause the cerebral cortex to send impulses to the motor center by way of the hypothalamus (see Chapter 3). The motor center then relays the impulses to the arterioles. The resulting vasoconstriction increases blood pressure. At the same time, the adrenal gland receives sympathetic impulses that cause it to release epinephrine and norepinephrine, both of which make the vasoconstriction last longer and help to maintain higher blood pressure levels.

Impulses from higher brain centers can also decrease stimulation of the vasomotor center. This would result in vasodilation and a fall in blood pressure.

Did you know?

How much of your blood supply do you think is normally present in different parts of your body? At any one time, about 5% of your blood is in your capillaries, 8% is in the heart, 12% is in the blood vessels in the lungs, 15% is in your arteries and arterioles, and 60% is in your veins and venules. It is easy to see why veins, especially those in the abdominal area and the skin, are called blood reservoirs.

Autoregulation of blood flow

There is another way your body regulates blood flow and blood pressure that is independent of the control of your vasomotor center. Autoregulation is your body's automatic adjustment of the flow of blood to a particular tissue in response to the special needs of that tissue.

Autoregulation can be stimulated by a physical condition. Take temperature, for example. When you are warm, your vessels automatically dilate to lower blood pressure. The reverse is also true—being cold causes vasoconstriction.

Chemical stimuli also result in autoregulation by causing the production of vasoactive factors, which are substances that can cause vasodilation or vasoconstriction. When your oxygen level is low, your cells produce chemicals that cause vasodilation of the arterioles in the immediate area. The resulting increase in blood flow restores oxygen levels to normal.

Other vasoactive factors produce vasoconstriction, resulting in decreased blood flow to tissue. Autoregulation is important for meeting the nutritional demands of active tissues such as muscle tissue.

Challenge of gravity

The fact that humans walk upright presents a considerable challenge to the cardiovascular system. Gravity presents two separate problems, both of which can have an effect on blood pressure and on fainting.

When humans stand or sit, their head is located above their heart. This means that the heart has to work against gravity in order to pump oxygen-rich blood up through the carotid arteries in your neck and into the arteries in your brain.

The same is true of the veins found in all parts of the body located below heart level. The flow of oxygen-poor blood through your veins back to the heart is affected by (1) the pumping action of your heart, (2) the speed of blood flow, (3) the contractions of your skeletal muscles, (4) the valves in your veins, and (5) your breathing. As you read, keep in mind that substances naturally move from an area of higher pressure to one of lower pressure.

Pumping action of the heart

The blood in the venules is under slightly higher pressure than blood that is in the right atrium, causing blood to move in the direction of the heart. Also, when the ventricles contract, the atrium above each ventricle becomes larger, decreasing its internal pressure and sucking in blood from the large veins emptying into it.

Speed of blood flow

The speed, or velocity, of blood flow depends on the size of the lumen of the blood vessel. Blood moves more quickly through larger arteries and more slowly through smaller arteries, arterioles, and capillaries. The speed of blood flow is slowest in your capillaries. As many capillaries join together to form venules and then veins, blood flow increases somewhat in speed as the vessels become larger.

Contractions of skeletal muscle and the valves in the veins

The contractions of your skeletal muscles work together with the system of valves in your veins to help you return oxygen-poor blood from your lower body to your heart. When your skeletal muscles contract, they press on veins passing through them and open the valves. This pressure pushes blood toward the heart—an action sometimes called "milking" (see Figure 4-7). When the skeletal muscles relax, the valves close to prevent blood from flowing back away from the heart.

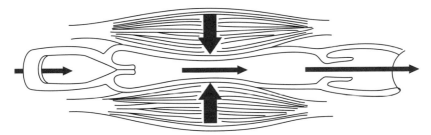

Figure 4-7 When the skeletal muscles contract, they press on veins passing through them and open the valves. This pressure pushes blood toward the heart—an action sometimes called "milking".

People who are bedridden do not often contract their muscles. As a result, the return of oxygen-poor blood to the heart is slower and the heart has to work harder in these individuals.

Breathing

Breathing is an important factor in returning blood to your heart. As you recall, your diaphragm is a muscle stretching across the inside of your body, separating your chest from your abdomen. When you breath in, your lungs expand and your diaphragm moves downward. This downward movement of the diaphragm makes the chest area larger, decreasing the pressure inside it. At the same time, inhaling causes the abdominal area to decrease in size, thereby increasing its internal pressure. As a result, when you breathe in, blood moves from the abdomen where pressure is higher upward into the chest area where pressure is lower.

What about when you breathe out? The changes in the pressures are reversed. As the diaphragm moves back upward, pressure is decreased in the abdomen and increased in the chest. Fortunately, the valves in the vein again come to the rescue, closing to prevent blood from flowing backward from the chest to the abdomen.

Looking forward . . .

The basic information on your nervous system and cardiovascular system provided in Chapters 3 and 4 should make it much easier to understand the various causes underlying the fainting phenomenon. In most cases, fainting results from a failure to compensate for the pooling of blood in the lower part of your body when you move from a lying position to a sitting or standing position. As you will see, any number of things that can go wrong, ultimately leading to the same result—a loss of consciousness.

The conditions discussed in Chapters 5 through 9 tend to have very technical names, containing long words and unfamiliar terms. Our use of these accepted names will help you recognize them when your doctor mentions them or when you hear or read about them.

Reference

Tortora GJ. *Introduction to the Human Body: The Essentials of Anatomy and Physiology*, 4th edition. Menlo Park, CA: Biological Sciences Textbooks, Inc., 1997.

Orthostatic intolerance and orthostatic (postural) hypotension

The term *orthostatic intolerance* is not exactly familiar to most people. What does it mean, anyway? The word orthostatic describes something that is caused by standing upright. Therefore, orthostatic intolerance is a general term referring to a cluster of symptoms that some people experience as the result of simply standing up.

As shown in Table 5-1, a large number of terms have been used to describe orthostatic intolerance over the years. As you continue reading, some of the terms in Table 5-1 will become more familiar since the various conditions discussed in this book are different forms of orthostatic intolerance.

The most common symptoms associated with orthostatic intolerance include (Low et al., 1995a)

- lightheadedness,
- weakness or tiredness,
- difficulty thinking and concentrating,
- blurred vision,
- tremulousness (feeling shaky),
- vertigo (a sensation of revolving or spinning motion, either of yourself or things around you),
- pallor (paleness or loss of skin color),
- anxiety,
- rapid heart rate or "heart palpitations" (feeling that your heart is beating quickly and forcefully or fluttering),
- clammy feeling, and
- nausea.

Some researchers have found it useful to set up a system of grading for orthostatic intolerance based on the symptoms associated with it. This system is given in Table 5-2.

Introducing orthostatic hypotension

Many of the underlying causes for orthostatic intolerance result in a condition called orthostatic hypotension (low blood pressure). Orthostatic, or postural, hypotension is a sudden drop in blood pressure resulting from your moving to an upright position or posture. This change in posture most often involves standing up from a squatting or sitting position. However, some people may experience symptoms of orthostatic hypotension when they sit up from a lying

Da Costa's syndrome
Hyperadrenergic orthostatic hypotension
Hyperadrenergic orthostatic tachycardia
Hyperdynamic beta-adrenergic state
Idiopathic hypovolemia
Idiopathic orthostatic intolerance
Idiopathic orthostatic tachycardia
Irritable heart
Mitral valve prolapse syndrome
Neurocirculatory asthenia
Orthostatic anemia
Orthostatic intolerance
Orthostatic tachycardia
Orthostatic tachycardia plus
Orthostatic tachycardia syndrome
Partial dysautonomia
Postural orthostatic tachycardia syndrome
Postural tachycardia syndrome
Soldier's heart
Sympathicotonic orthostatic hypotension
Sympathotonic orthostatic hypotension
Vasoregulatory asthenia

Table 5-1 Various names used to describe orthostatic intolerance.

Table 5-2 Grading of orthostatic intolerance.

Grades	Associated symptoms
Grade 0	Normal orthostatic tolerance
Grade 1	Orthostatic symptoms are rare or only occur under conditions of increased orthostatic stress (such as standing for long periods, eating a meal, exerting yourself, or heat stress). Symptoms may vary with time, circumstances, and the amount of blood volume present. You are able to stand more than 15 minutes on most occasions. You typically have unrestricted activities of daily living.
Grade 2	Orthostatic symptoms develop at least once a week. These symptoms commonly develop with orthostatic stress. You are able to stand more than 5 minutes on most occasions. You typically have some limitation in activities of daily living.
Grade 3	Orthostatic symptoms develop on most occasions and are regularly intensified by orthostatic stresses (see above). You are able to stand more than 1 minute on most occasions. You typically have some limitation in activities of daily living.
Grade 4	Orthostatic symptoms are consistently present. You are able to stand less than 1 minute on most occasions. You are seriously disabled, being bedridden or wheelchair-bound due to orthostatic intolerance. Fainting or symptoms typically preceding fainting (presyncope) are common if you try to stand up.

Adapted from Low et al., 1995b.

position such as sitting up on the side of the bed. Orthostatic hypotension may, but does not always, result in a faint.

Did you know?

Doctors typically use the word "syncope" to indicate a faint. You will see this word used as part of the official names of several of the underlying causes for fainting discussed in this book.

Before taking a closer look at orthostatic hypotension, first consider all of the processes involved every time you simply stand up.

Assuming an upright posture

A lot of things happen very quickly in your body after you stand up from a sitting or squatting position. These changes in posture bring gravity into play in your blood supply… in a big way.

Effects of posture on your blood pressure

Normally, about one-fourth of your blood is in your chest area. However, when you change your posture to become upright, gravity quickly pulls about 17 fluid ounces (500 ml or more than 2 cups) of blood down into your abdomen and legs. When all of your systems are working properly, about half of this blood is moved back into your upper body very quickly—within seconds. In a normal situation, your blood pressure will begin to stabilize within a minute or less of your assuming an upright posture.

As fast as this response may be, your heart will have beaten several times during the precious seconds when the blood supply in the upper body is lower than normal. What exactly happens? For one thing, as a result of the blood pooling, your systemic circulation will have less blood available to be returned to the right atrium of your heart. Less blood getting to the right atrium translates to a right ventricle that is not able to fill entirely with blood before it contracts. The fact that the ventricle was only partially filled reduces the stroke volume—the amount of blood ejected out of the ventricle and into the artery in a minute—by about 40%. So less blood is sent to your lungs to pick up oxygen.

A few heartbeats later, these same reactions also occur in the left atrium and ventricle. Why the short delay? When the right side of the heart first begins to experience a reduced blood return, the left side of the heart is still receiving the normal amount of blood from your lungs—your pulmonary circulation. Once the heart has beaten a few times, however, the left side of your heart also experiences the reduced blood flow.

But the effects do not stop there. The reduced amount of blood being pumped from your ventricles causes the blood pressure in your arteries to fall. This decrease in blood pressure alerts your baroreceptors. Recall from Chapter 4, when blood pressure is abnormally high, baroreceptors send impulses to stimulate an inhibitory response in the cardiovascular center. This leads to an increase in parasympathetic impulses that inhibit heart function, resulting in a lower heart rate and decreased force of contraction. (See Chapter 3 for information on the autonomic nervous system, or ANS.)

On the other hand, when baroreceptors sense a fall in blood pressure, they stop sending impulses to stimulate an inhibitory response. This allows sympathetic impulses to dominate, ultimately resulting in increased heart rate and stronger contractions, leading to greater cardiac output. Sympathetic impulses also cause constriction of your blood vessels. All of these actions help raise your blood pressure back to normal levels.

In addition, there are other receptors—called mechanoreceptors—in the atria and ventricles of the heart and in the pulmonary arteries leading to the lungs. These receptors are sensitive to being stretched, such as when the chambers of the heart are filled with blood. Mechanoreceptors usually send continuous messages to that part of the cardiovascular center controlling the sympathetic division of the ANS. These messages cause the sympathetic responses that result in constriction of your blood vessels to be inhibited.

When there is less blood entering the heart, however, there is less stretching of the mechanoreceptors. This normally causes a decrease in the inhibitory messages sent to the sympathetic division. The resulting increase in sympathetic impulses causes vasoconstriction, which raises blood pressure. All of these early responses typically increase your heart rate by 10–15 beats per minute and your diastolic blood pressure by 10 mm Hg.

But that is not all. You also have other types of responses to your temporary fall in blood pressure. For example, if your body interprets the lowered blood pressure as being severe enough, your kidneys may secrete the enzyme renin. Renin is able to increase blood pressure by starting a series of activities that ultimately lead to the constriction of your arteries and the retention of fluid by your kidneys, which increases your blood volume.

Did you know?

Renin does not act directly on the blood vessels or kidneys. Here is the way it actually works: Renin is an enzyme that converts angiotensinogen (a large protein produced by the liver) to angiotensin I in your bloodstream. Then, as angiotensin I passes through your lungs, it is converted to the active hormone angiotensin II. Angiotensin II causes constriction of your arterioles, helping to raise your blood pressure. Angiotensin II also stimulates the adrenal glands to secrete aldosterone, a hormone that causes your kidneys to retain sodium and water, which also results in higher blood pressure.

Blood pressure and your brain

Meanwhile, what is happening to the blood flow to your brain while your cardiovascular and nervous systems are trying to reestablish normal blood pressure levels? As was mentioned previously, your brain uses about one-fifth of all the oxygen required by your body. Therefore, the brain has special mechanisms that allow it to protect its precious oxygen supply during swings in blood pressure that may occur throughout the day. Even when the blood pressure in the rest of the body is quite low, the blood flow to the brain usually stays fairly constant. If blood pressure goes up, the arterioles in the brain constrict. When blood pressure drops, the arterioles in the brain typically dilate or expand.

Most people are unaware of all these internal shifts and adjustments every time they rise to a standing (or even sitting) position. However, not everyone is able to counteract the effects of gravity on blood flow.

What happens in orthostatic hypotension?

Orthostatic hypotension is not a disease, as such, but represents an inability to regulate blood pressure quickly in response to postural changes. People with orthostatic hypotension are not able to compensate for the blood pooling in their lower body—primarily in the veins of their abdomen and legs—when they assume an upright position.

Did you know?

The "official" definition for orthostatic hypotension is a reduction of systolic blood pressure of at least 20 mm Hg or diastolic pressure of at least 10 mm Hg within 3 minutes of standing. A few people, however, may not experience the fall in blood pressure until they have been standing for at least 10 minutes. Therefore, some doctors consider a practical definition for orthostatic hypotension to be any drop in blood pressure on standing that results in symptoms.

Keep in mind that even when the heart receives enough blood and blood pressure is normal, it still has to pump against gravity to deliver blood to the brain, which is usually situated above heart level. When too little blood gets back to the heart, a reduced amount of blood is available to be pumped to the brain. Without sufficient oxygen-rich blood, the brain can temporarily cease to function, causing unconsciousness.

Common causes of orthostatic hypotension

Orthostatic hypotension can have many underlying causes. For convenience, the major causes of orthostatic hypotension are often divided into those that are neurogenic, or related to the nervous system, and those that are nonneurogenic.

Neurogenic causes of orthostatic hypotension

You have already seen how important the ANS is to your ability to regain normal blood pressures after you stand up. Therefore, it should come as no surprise that orthostatic hypotension can be due to disorders of the ANS—either primary or secondary to another disease. Since the ANS controls heart rate, people with neurogenic orthostatic hypotension do not experience a normal increase in heart rate as their blood pressure falls.

The causes of neurogenic orthostatic hypotension are considered to be primary when they result from some type of ANS failure. In fact, orthostatic hypotension is often a sign that the ANS is not functioning properly. Therefore, orthostatic hypotension is a common symptom of many diseases, disorders, or conditions associated with problems of the nerves or the nervous system.

Secondary causes of neurogenic orthostatic hypotension can include physical deformities of the nerves or nervous system or abnormalities in some of the enzymes necessary for normal ANS function. However, the most common type of secondary cause is a group of diseases and syndromes that result in malfunctions of the nervous system. In this case, the disease or condition causes an injury to part of the brain, spinal cord, or peripheral nervous system (PNS), resulting in problems with blood pressure control. Examples of diseases that damage the central nervous system (CNS) include multiple sclerosis and Parkinson's disease. The most common disorders of the PNS that result in orthostatic hypotension include diabetes mellitus, Guillain-Barré syndrome, and polyneuropathy (a generalized disorder of the peripheral nerves) due to alcoholism (Engstrom and Aminoff, 1997).

Table 5-3 lists some of the more common primary and secondary causes of neurogenic orthostatic hypotension. A description of all these diseases or conditions is beyond the scope of this book.

In many instances, the underlying cause of orthostatic hypotension may not be treatable. When this is the case, your doctor will most likely prescribe treatments to help combat the orthostatic hypotension itself—treating the symptom rather than the disease causing it.

Nonneurogenic causes of orthostatic hypotension

When orthostatic hypotension has a nonneurogenic cause, the drop in blood pressure typically is accompanied by a normal increase in heart rate. This increase in heart rate, which may exceed 30 beats per minute, may help compensate for the fall in blood pressure.

Nonneurogenic causes for orthostatic hypotension can include conditions in which the heart does not pump properly, a reduction in blood volume, or an increased pooling of blood in the veins in the lower part of the body. In addition, orthostatic hypotension is often a side effect of medications, especially in older individuals.

Table 5-3 Selected disorders of the nervous system that may result in orthostatic hypotension and fainting.

Primary failure of the ANS
Pure autonomic failure
Multiple system atrophy (Shy-Drager syndrome)
Subacute malfunctioning of the ANS

Secondary autonomic failure
Central nervous system
  Brain and brainstem
    Age-related
    Multiple sclerosis
    Brain tumors
    Parkinson's disease
  Spinal cord
    Transverse myelitus
    Syringomyelia
    Spinal tumor
    Tabes dorsalis

Peripheral Nervous System
  Diabetes mellitus
  Guillain-Barré syndrome
  HIV infection
  Amyloidosis
  Porphyria
  Dopamine-β-hydroxylase deficiency
  Polyneuropathy (generalized disorder of the peripheral nerves) due to alcoholism

---

Adapted from Engstrom and Martin, 1998.

Pump failure

When the heart fails to pump properly, you cannot maintain a normal blood pressure. Here are some conditions in which the heart does not pump properly and which can result in orthostatic hypotension and, possibly, fainting:

Myocardial infarction—A myocardial infarction (MI) is the technical term for a heart attack. As you recall from Chapter 4, the myocardium is the muscular middle layer of heart muscle. An infarction is an area of tissue that is damaged as the result of blood flow being cut off. In the case of an MI, part of myocardium, which is responsible for the heart contracting, is damaged by a loss of blood and does not function properly. This can potentially reduce the heart's ability to pump blood throughout the body.

Myocarditis—Myocarditis is an inflammation of the myocardium of the heart. As in the case of an MI, myocarditis can negatively affect the ability of the heart to pump blood effectively.

Constrictive pericarditis—The heart is enclosed in a loose-fitting sac called the pericardium. Pericarditis is an inflammation of the pericardium. This condition can lead to a buildup of fluid or blood in the space between the pericardium and the heart. Since the pericardium cannot stretch, this fluid buildup can put pressure on the heart, limiting its ability to pump properly.

Aortic stenosis—Stenosis refers to a narrowing of a passage or duct. Therefore, aortic stenosis is an abnormal narrowing of the aortic valve, that is, the semilunar valve between the left ventricle of the heart and the ascending aorta (see Chapter 4). This condition limits the amount of blood that the left ventricle can eject with each contraction, reducing the blood available to be circulated to the brain and other parts of the body in systemic circulation.

Tachyarrhythmia—Tachycardia is a rapid heart rate, that is, a heart rate above 100 beats per minute (in an adult). When tachycardia occurs, the ventricles do not have time to fill properly before ejecting blood out into your circulatory systems. Arrhythmia refers to an irregularity in the force or rhythm of your heartbeat. Putting these two terms together, tachyarrhythmia describes a heartbeat that is both rapid and irregular, causing a reduction in normal blood flow from the heart to the rest of the body.

Bradyarrhythmia—Bradycardia is a slow heart rate—usually under 60 beats per minute. Therefore, bradyarrhythmia is a disturbance in the heart's normal rhythm that results in a slow, irregular heart rate. Here again, this can cause too little blood to be ejected, thereby lowering your blood pressure when you stand up.

Low blood volume

Any condition or situation that substantially decreases the amount of blood you have in circulation can potentially cause orthostatic hypotension and fainting. Here are some examples of situations or conditions that can result in a low blood volume.

Hemorrhage—Hemorrhage is any excessive loss of blood from your blood vessels. If the blood loss is large enough, it can result in a drop in blood pressure, which can cause orthostatic hypotension.

Dehydration—Dehydration refers to a large loss of water from your body. For example, some people do not consume enough fluid to offset the amount being lost in urine. The risk of dehydration increases with the use of diuretics ("water pills"), which increase urination. At times, fluid loss may be the result of vomiting, diarrhea, or excessive sweating. Whatever causes the fluid loss, it can reduce the volume of blood available for circulation and lead to orthostatic hypotension.

Burns—When body tissues are burned, fluid leaks from the surrounding blood vessels. If the burn covers a large area, a much greater amount of fluid can be lost from blood, resulting in a drop in blood volume and blood pressure. This situation can potentially lead to orthostatic hypotension.

Straining—Do you ever feel yourself straining when you lift something heavy—or sometimes when you go to the bathroom? Did you know that this straining may cause orthostatic hypotension? Straining when you lift something heavy, urinate, pass stool, or even cough can raise the pressure in your chest area. This may potentially reduce the amount of blood being returned from your abdomen and legs through your chest to your heart. In some people, this reduction in blood return is substantial enough to drop blood pressure and increase the likelihood of orthostatic hypotension and even fainting.

Kidney diseases that cause salt loss—Your kidneys are largely responsible for fluid balance in the body. For example, they regulate the amount of fluid and sodium in your system.

Sodium is a mineral that has many vital functions in your body. In addition to helping regulate fluid balance, sodium plays an important role in the transmission of nerve impulses in nervous and muscle tissue. Your kidneys normally retain sodium when you cut down on your intake of salt and other sodium-containing compounds. When you have excess sodium, your kidneys excrete it and the fluid that goes with it in urine.

Some kidney diseases cause you to lose too much sodium, which results in an abnormally large amount of urine being excreted from the body. This lowers blood volume and blood pressure, possibly causing orthostatic hypotension.

Insufficient functioning of the adrenal gland—You have two adrenal glands, one located above each kidney. The adrenal glands produce several substances that play a role in the mechanism by which your body controls blood pressure. For example, the adrenal glands produce the hormone neurotransmitters epinephrine and norepinephrine, which affect heart rate and blood pressure. Your adrenal glands also produce substances called mineralocorticoids (see Chapter 11) that control the body's use of sodium and potassium, thereby affecting fluid balance in your body.

Diabetes insipidus—When you hear the word diabetes, you usually think of diabetes mellitus. However, there is also a condition called diabetes insipidus. Diabetes insipidus typically develops as the result of a decreased production of the hormone vasopressin. Vasopressin is an antidiuretic hormone, that is, it prevents too much urine from being excreted. Therefore, when the level of vasopressin is low, you excrete more urine, potentially reducing the volume of fluid in your body. Sometimes diabetes insipidus can occur when there are normal levels of vasopressin but the kidneys do not have a normal response to this hormone.

Venous pooling

Venous pooling is an excessive amount of blood settling in the large veins in the lower part of the body, your abdomen and legs. When this occurs, less blood is available to return to the heart through the venules and veins, which results in a lower blood pressure. There are various factors that can increase venous pooling:

Alcohol—Alcohol can cause a fall in blood pressure when you are supine, that is, lying on your back. This makes you much more likely to experience orthostatic hypotension when you stand, dropping your blood pressure to levels low enough to cause symptoms. Research has also shown that alcohol causes dilation—enlargement—of an artery in the abdomen (superior mesenteric artery), which could contribute to lowering of blood pressure (Chaudhuri et al., 1994).

Postprandial hypotension—Postprandial means "after a meal." Postprandial hypotension is often defined as a decrease in systolic blood pressure of 20 mm Hg or more within 2 hours of starting a meal.

After you eat, there normally is a pooling of blood in the abdominal region due to the increased activity of your digestive organs. The body usually responds by increasing the activity of the sympathetic nervous system, which results in a slight increase in heart rate and cardiac output to compensate for the pooling effect. In people who develop postprandial hypotension, however, there is not adequate compensation and blood pressure drops, leading to symptoms that often include fainting. Postprandial hypotension is especially common in older people who have high blood pressure.

Vigorous exercise—Vigorous exercise results in the dilation of blood vessels located in the skeletal muscles being worked. This may temporarily remove enough blood from general circulation to drop blood pressure, leading to orthostatic hypotension.

Heat—Heat expands blood vessels in the lower body, causing them to hold more blood. The reduced return of blood to the heart can lead to orthostatic hypotension. The heat can be from hot weather—especially if it is hot and humid—or from a heating system within your home or another building. Hot showers and baths also dilate blood vessels, as does having a fever.

Lying or standing for long periods—It is easy to see that standing in one position for a long period allows gravity to have its greatest effect on your blood volume, pulling it away from your head and into your lower body. As you may recall from Chapter 4, contractions of the skeletal muscles in your legs compress the veins, helping them transport blood from your lower body to your heart. But, when you have been lying down or standing still in one position for a long period of time, these muscles have not been able to do their job. This can contribute to the pooling of blood in your lower body.

Sepsis—Sepsis is an infection of a wound or tissue caused by bacteria and leading to the formation of pus. Sepsis is often accompanied by a fever. The increase of blood flow to an infected area plus the vasodilation resulting from a fever may contribute to venous pooling.

Medications

There are a number of drugs that can cause orthostatic hypotension. Some drugs, such as diuretics, decrease your blood volume by increasing the amount of fluid loss in urine you excrete through your kidneys. Other drugs may act as vasodilators, expanding the size of the blood vessels in your lower body and making it more difficult to return sufficient blood back to the heart. By the way, vasodilators also act as mild diuretics, increasing fluid loss.

Make sure your doctor knows about any medication you are taking. You may never suspect that the drug can be contributing to your fainting problem.

Table 5-4 Drugs that may cause orthostatic hypotension.

These Drugs...	Are Commonly Used...
Antihypertensive agents	To reduce high blood pressure, which can potentially cause orthostatic hypotension
Diuretics ("water pills")	To increase elimination of water and salt by the kidneys, thereby reducing high blood pressure or to decrease retention of excess fluid ("bloating")
Angiotensin-converting enzyme inhibitors	To suppress the conversion of renin-angiotensin I to angiotensin II, thereby preventing constriction of your arterioles and retention of sodium and fluid in your kidneys
Alpha-blocking agents	To cause dilation of peripheral blood vessels, which lowers peripheral resistance and reduces blood pressure
Beta-blocking agents	To block the stimulating effect of epinephrine on the heart, thereby reducing heart rate and the force of heart contractions
Calcium channel-blocking agents	To block the entry of calcium into smooth muscle, resulting in relaxation of heart muscle, dilation of heart and peripheral arteries, and slowing of heart rate
Other vasodilator drugs (nitrates, hydralazine)	To dilate or widen the arteries in the heart and peripheral blood vessels
Other agents	
Tricyclic antidepressants	To treat depression
Phenothiazines	As an antipsychotic agent or, occasionally, to control vomiting
Bromocriptine	To treat Parkinson's disease
CNS sedatives (barbiturates and opiates)	To relieve pain

Table 5-4 shows the general types of drugs that may have orthostatic hypotension as a side effect.

Symptoms of orthostatic hypotension

Not everyone who has orthostatic hypotension experiences symptoms. However, as you might expect, those individuals who do develop symptoms on assuming an erect posture typically report
- lightheadedness,
- faintness,
- blurred vision or even loss of vision,
- weakness,
- difficulty in mental processes,
- unsteadiness after standing or walking,

- dizziness,
- fatigue,
- nausea,
- heart palpitations,
- tremulousness or feeling shaky,
- headache, and
- neck pain (described as "coat-hanger"-shaped pain).

The first six symptoms often occur together. They tend to be worse in the morning, affecting you when you initially get out of bed. Symptoms may also be worse in people who have been lying down for long periods, are in a hot and humid environment (such as hot weather, central heating, or a hot bath), have eaten a heavy meal, or have just exercised.

Experiencing a faint due to orthostatic hypotension

Remember that not everyone who has orthostatic hypotension faints. But, what actually does happen when orthostatic hypotension causes you to faint? This type of fainting episode typically has three phases:

- presyncope ("before syncope"),
- actual loss of consciousness, and
- postsyncope ("after syncope").

Presyncope

Presyncope, or aura, is the period just before you lose consciousness. It may last up to half a minute or so and can occur while you are standing or walking. In a fainting episode, you may stumble and fall to your knees before losing consciousness. As you might expect, the symptom list is very similar to the one for orthostatic hypotension. Symptoms that typically warn of an approaching faint may include

- weakness,
- dizziness and lightheadedness,
- blurring, dimming, or loss of vision,
- "tunnel" vision (ability to see only things directly in front of you—in a narrow tunnel—but not off to the side),
- sweating,
- reduced hearing,
- becoming pale,
- nausea,
- abdominal discomfort,
- vertigo,
- "palpitations",
- headache,
- vomiting, and
- inability to concentrate or focus your thoughts.

In one large study, the researchers found that the most common symptoms occurring during presyncope were weakness (44%), dizziness (44%), blurred vision (33%), sweating (33%), nausea (29%), and abdominal discomfort (11%) (Linzer et al., 1990). As unpleasant as these symptoms may be, they can provide a chance for you to take certain steps before you lose consciousness. Lying down, for example, may prevent or lessen the severity of an episode and should at least protect you from injuries due to a fall.

Loss of consciousness

Most people who faint do not remember losing consciousness. The people around the person who has fainted commonly are called upon to describe what actually happened. Bystanders report that unconscious individuals typically are pale or ashen. Their skin is cold and they are sweating heavily. Their pupils may be dilated. In a few instances, people who faint may urinate or lose control of their bowels.

Observers tend to be most impressed by the convulsions, which usually, but not always, begin after the person is unconscious. The unconscious person may experience a long contraction (tonic) or an alternating contraction and relaxation (clonic) of the muscles in the arms and legs with a raising and backward throw of the head.

Postsyncope

People with orthostatic hypotension who faint are usually unconscious for a relatively short time, some for only seconds. As a rule, they recover rapidly from a faint and do not suffer from confusion. However, these individuals may complain of nervousness, headache, and/or nausea after they have regained consciousness.

Looking forward...

This information on orthostatic hypotension—in general and as a cause of fainting—provides the basis for the chapters that follow.

Discussing every single possible cause of fainting is beyond the scope of this book. However, this chapter and the next four chapters should make you familiar with the most common causes of fainting.

References

Chaudhuri KR, Maule S, Thomaides T, et al. Alcohol ingestion lowers supine blood pressure, causes splanchnic vasodilation, and worsens postural hypotension in primary autonomic failure. *Journal of Neurology* 1994;241:145–152.

Engstrom JW, Aminoff MJ. Evaluation and treatment of orthostatic hypotension. *American Family Physician* 1997;56:1378–1384.

Engstrom JW, Martin JP. Disorders of the autonomic nervous system. In: Fauci AS, ed. *Harrison's Principles of Internal Medicine*. New York: McGraw-Hill, 1998.

Grubb BP. Dysautonomic (orthostatic) syncope. In: Grubb BP, Olshansky B, eds. *Syncope: Mechanisms and Management*. Malden MA, Blackwell/Futura Publishing Company, Inc., 2005:72–91.

Linzer M, Felder A, Hackel A, et al. Psychiatric syncope. *Psychomatics* 1990;31:181–188.

Low PA, Opfer-Gehrking TL, McPhee BR, et al. Prospective evaluation of clinical characteristics of orthostatic hypotension. *Mayo Clinic Proceedings* 1995a;70:617–622.

Low PA, Opfer-Gehrking TL, Textor SC, et al. Postural tachycardia syndrome (POTS). *Neurology* 1995b; 45(Suppl 5):S19–S25.

Streeten DHP, Anderson GH Jr. Delayed orthostatic intolerance. *Archives of Internal Medicine* 1992; 152:1066–1072.

CHAPTER 6

Neurocardiogenic syncope

The parts of the word *neurocardiogenic* hint at its meaning. *Neuro* refers to the nervous system and cardio refers to the heart. The suffix *genic* means "produced by." And syncope is fainting. So, putting it all together, neurocardiogenic syncope is fainting produced by something going wrong between your heart and nervous system. Neurocardiogenic syncope usually, but not always, occurs when you assume an upright position, or posture. People with neurocardiogenic syncope often have no evidence of heart disease or of abnormalities in the heart's conduction system.

Basics of neurocardiogenic syncope

Neurocardiogenic syncope is the most common type of fainting phenomenon. It has been estimated that neurocardiogenic mechanisms may be partly or totally responsible for 50–80% of all fainting episodes (reviewed in Olshansky, 2005). Although researchers have not established the exact mechanism in neurocardiogenic syncope, they have a general idea of what happens.

Mechanoreceptors misfire

Go back to the sequence of events that occurs when you move to a sitting or standing position (see Chapter 5). First, gravity causes venous pooling— an increase in the amount of blood drawn downward into the large veins in your abdomen and legs. When venous pooling occurs in someone with neurocardiogenic syncope, there is a difference in the way the heart responds to the reduced amount of blood being returned to it and the way these responses are translated into action.

As you may recall from the previous chapter, there are mechanoreceptors in the atria and ventricles of the heart that normally respond to being stretched by the chamber being filled with blood. As long as the mechanoreceptors keep sending messages to the brain, the cardiovascular center continues to trigger the sympathetic responses that inhibit the constriction of your blood vessels.

When the left ventricle does not have sufficient blood to fill it to capacity, it responds by contracting much more forcefully. This is the heart's way of trying to raise your blood pressure. In someone with neurocardiogenic syncope, however, these strong contractions activate a large number of the mechanoreceptors that normally only respond to being stretched. Therefore, even though you have less blood present in the left ventricle and being ejected out of the heart, the mechanoreceptors respond as if the ventricle is actually overfilled. This means that the mechanoreceptors send messages to the sympathetic division of the autonomic nervous system (ANS) indicating that your blood pressure is actually high—hypertension. In response to this faulty message, the cardiovascular center reduces certain sympathetic impulses, which results in a slower heart rate and vasodilation—both of which lower blood pressure even further.

Research studies suggest that parasympathetic impulses to the heart, which cause a lower heart rate and strength of contraction, do increase somewhat during a faint. However, the primary cause of someone with neurocardiogenic syncope losing consciousness appears to be low blood pressure due to vasodilation, which is under the direction of sympathetic impulses.

Serotonin connection

Although a lot of people have become familiar with serotonin, not everyone understands what it is and how it works in the body. Serotonin is a neurotransmitter found in the central nervous system (CNS).

How do neurotransmitters work? If you recall from Chapter 3, impulses are transmitted across the tiny gap (synapse) between nerve cells, or neurons, by chemical substances called neurotransmitters. First, the neurotransmitter is released from sacs at the end of an axon on one neuron. Next, it travels over the synaptic space between the neurons. Then, it is picked up by a receptor on the dendrite located at the end of the next neuron in line. Dendrites have different kinds of receptors because a single receptor typically responds only to a particular neurotransmitter (or group of similar substances). However, a neurotransmitter may be able to attach to more than one type of receptor. For example, there are at least 14 types of serotonin receptors in the CNS. Each receptor is responsible for receiving and passing on an impulse that ultimately results in a different function. Think of it as a key: the neurotransmitter (and related substances) fitting into a lock or series of locks—the receptors—that only it will fit. Which neurotransmitter is produced and present in the synapse determines whether a nerve impulse passes from one neuron to another or from a neuron to a tissue.

As a rule, serotonin causes the inhibition of a nerve impulse. Therefore, production of serotonin and its release into the synapse inhibits the passage of impulses from one neuron to the next. Studies in animals have shown that the withdrawal of sympathetic impulses is directly due to a higher level of serotonin being present in the CNS, the brain, and spinal cord. Researchers are currently studying this phenomenon. The application of this information about serotonin will become clear when you learn about different drug treatments that are sometimes used for neurocardiogenic syncope.

Response of the brain

In people with neurocardiogenic syncope, the reduction in blood flow to the brain causes a sudden constriction instead of an enlargement of the arteries.

This results in both an increase in the speed of the blood flow and a loss of blood pressure in the narrowed segment of artery. The result is that the brain does not receive the oxygen it needs. This abrupt vasoconstriction appears to occur before, and possibly contributes to, the actual fainting episode.

In addition, a few people with chronic fainting problems appear to develop vasoconstriction of the arteries in their brain even when their blood pressure and heart rate are normal.

Did you know?

Do not get confused if you run across the term "vasovagal syncope". It actually is the same as neurocardiogenic syncope, which has generally become the preferred term.

Potential triggers for neurocardiogenic syncope

Changing your posture—sitting or standing up—is not the only possible trigger for neurocardiogenic syncope. Any situation that results in a decreased blood flow to the heart could potentially cause the left ventricle to contract too strongly and trigger the faulty mechanoreceptors to send an incorrect message to the brain.

Therefore, other potential triggers for neurocardiogenic syncope may include any condition that even temporarily results in low blood pressure.

Reduction in blood volume
A severe reduction in blood volume causes a drop in blood pressure that could potentially lead to neurocardiogenic syncope. The most obvious cause of a low blood volume is hemorrhage—excessive bleeding. If the reduction in blood volume occurs as the result of fluid lost in diarrhea or vomiting, the fainting episode may be an isolated incident and never happen again.

Postprandial state
As already mentioned in the previous chapter, postprandial simply means "after a meal." In some people, eating causes a fall in blood pressure, usually peaking from 30 to 60 minutes after completion of the meal. Unfortunately, the timing is just right to affect diners as they are getting up from the table.

Vigorous exercise in a warm environment
People who exercise vigorously on a warm day (or in any warm environment) run the risk of becoming dehydrated. This excessive fluid loss from sweating may be accompanied by salt loss, which can also cause an increase in your fluid loss in urine. If you lose too much fluid and reduce your blood volume, the result is low blood pressure, which may lead to the neurocardiogenic response and to fainting in susceptible people. Some studies investigating

neurocardiogenic syncope related to exercise suggest that the primary under-lying cause is vasodilation when the arteries should properly be constricting to help maintain normal blood pressure.

Sodium restriction and/or diuretic use

When people follow a diet that is reduced in sodium, the purpose usually is to increase their fluid loss in urine. Diuretics are substances, usually medications, that cause the kidneys to excrete more fluid as urine. Doctors often prescribe both dietary sodium restriction and diuretics for blood pressure control. How-ever, too much fluid can be lost at times, resulting in low blood pressure and, potentially, fainting.

Emotional and/or stressful situations

Sometimes emotional and/or stressful situations can trigger neurocardiogenic syncope. These emotions might include responses to real or imagined danger, fear, or anxiety. Some people about to get an injection—a shot—may faint from the anxiety of just seeing a needle or from the sight of blood.

Other causes

Alcohol may also increase your likelihood of neurocardiogenic responses that lead to low blood pressure and loss of consciousness. And jet lag has been known to cause susceptible people to develop problems with low blood pres-sure and fainting. Whatever the cause, when blood pressure drops low enough to prevent sufficient blood from being circulated to the brain, the result is a faint.

Experiencing neurocardiogenic syncope

The three phases that are typical of a fainting episode—presyncope, loss of consciousness, and postsyncope—were reviewed in the previous chapter. However, many people with neurocardiogenic syncope do not experience presyncope. This is especially true of older people. Instead, individuals with neurocardiogenic syncope may have what is called a "drop attack," which means that they lose consciousness without any warning. As you might imag-ine, a person who abruptly loses consciousness has no time to take defensive measures. This type of fall can lead to serious injuries, particularly in older individuals. Do not underestimate the possible danger associated with falls. They can cause serious injuries, lead to disability, and even result in death. Although most of the time people are unconscious for only a short period—even seconds—some individuals may be unconscious up to 15 minutes.

When people with neurocardiogenic syncope do experience presyncope, it is liable to include symptoms similar to those for orthostatic hypotension, including

• weakness,
• dizziness and lightheadedness,
• blurred vision,
• sweating,

- nausea,
- abdominal discomfort,
- vertigo,
- "palpitations",
- headache,
- vomiting,
- disorientation,
- difficulty in speaking clearly or coherently, and
- narrowed visual field or "tunnel vision".

There are other people who experience the drop in blood pressure and show symptoms of too little oxygen reaching the brain without ever completely losing consciousness. These individuals are likely to go to a doctor with complaints of severe dizziness, lightheadedness, vertigo, and disturbance of their sense of balance (equilibrium). It is fairly common for these people to be referred to a doctor who specializes in evaluating and treating conditions of the ear, nose, and throat (otolaryngologist). This type of specialist may or may not recognize the actual root of the problem.

Who develops neurocardiogenic syncope?

Neurocardiogenic syncope is the most common cause of fainting in younger people but not in older individuals. In most cases, younger people, including adolescents, tend to have classic neurocardiogenic syncope, pretty much the way it was previously described. (See Chapter 9 for more information about fainting in younger and older individuals.)

When neurocardiogenic syncope develops in adolescents, it is often following a rapid growth spurt. Young women tend to experience episodes more often around the time of their menstrual period, especially during the premenstrual days. Even when the fainting episodes are frequent and severe, they often spontaneously disappear by the time the teen has reached his or her mid-twenties. However, women who suffered from neurocardiogenic syncope in adolescence that later disappeared may experience recurrences of this condition during pregnancy and/or immediately after the baby is born.

Researchers have identified certain individuals who faint in response to a number of stimuli. They are sometimes described as having a "hypersensitive" ANS. When their heartbeat becomes so slowed that it stops—asystole—for prolonged periods during a faint or during tilt-table testing (see Chapter 10), they are said to have the "malignant" form of neurocardiogenic syncope, which can mimic or may lead to sudden death. These individuals may require cardiopulmonary resuscitation to restart their breathing.

Some research suggests that people with recurring neurocardiogenic syncope are more likely than the general public to also have certain psychiatric conditions. These psychiatric disorders include major depression, panic disorder, and somatization disorder. Somatization disorder may be less familiar to you than panic disorder and depression. Basically, it is a condition in which a person reports many physical symptoms, usually involving a variety of organ systems, for which the doctor can find no physical cause.

Other studies indicate that people with neurocardiogenic syncope have an increased incidence of physical conditions with a psychological component. For example, individuals with neurocardiogenic syncope are more likely to suffer from migraine and chronic vascular headaches, indigestion, peptic ulcer disease, and unstable bowel syndrome.

And, at the other end of the health scale, some highly trained and recreational athletes experience exercise-related neurocardiogenic syncope during and following physical activity. Although the underlying cause has not been definitely established, the response during exercise is thought to be due to a greater degree of expansion in the blood vessels. Either they expand too much or are unable to constrict enough to raise blood pressure. When the fainting episode occurs after exercise, it is thought to be primarily due to a slowing of the heart rate.

Did you know?

Some animals experience a response similar to neurocardiogenic syncope. When certain animals are cornered, they have a particular type of "fight or flight" response. If they are trapped and cannot run away, they may exhibit a slower heart rate and loss of arterial constriction due to a reduction in sympathetic activity. They become totally motionless—actually playing "dead" until the danger has passed.

Putting it all together

Keep in mind that "classic" neurocardiogenic syncope typically includes both low blood pressure (hypotension) and a slower heart rate (bradycardia). Normally, a drop in blood pressure would signal your brain to speed up your heart rate to try to get your blood pressure back to normal levels. And this increase in heart rate does initially occur. However, the strong contractions of the ventricle walls cause a response in the mechanoreceptors, which misinterpret what is happening and send a message to your brain that your blood pressure is actually high. In response, the sympathetic portion of your cardiovascular center reduces its impulses to the heart and the parasympathetic division increases its impulses—both of which cause your heart rate to slow down. At the same time, the sympathetic division also reduces its impulses to your blood vessels, causing them to dilate. In fact, it is the enlargement of your blood vessels that is considered the primary cause of the continued low blood pressure.

When blood pressure falls low enough, the brain is no longer able to compensate and keep its blood flow constant. Once the oxygen supply to the brain is decreased for a long enough period, you will experience symptoms, including a temporary loss of consciousness—the faint.

Do not underestimate the seriousness of neurocardiogenic syncope. In addition to the injuries that can occur during a faint, some people experience potentially dangerous irregularities in their heart rate during an episode of neurocardiogenic syncope. There are instances of people being tested for neurocardiogenic syncope who had their hearts completely stop contracting—asystole (meaning without systole). If this condition is not promptly remedied, it can be fatal. Asystole also may degenerate into ventricular fibrillation—a rapid twitching of individual muscle fibers in which the muscular wall of the ventricle is unable to contract as a whole, resulting in a loss of pulse. Ventricular fibrillation is often fatal.

Looking forward . . .

Chapter 7 provides a brief look at postural tachycardia syndrome (POTS). POTS is another cause of fainting, this time associated with a fast heart rate.

References

Grubb BP. Neurocardiogenic syncope. In: Grubb BP, Olshansky B, eds. *Syncope: Mechanisms and Management*. Malden MA: Blackwell/Futura Publishing Co., Inc., 2005:47–71.

Kosinski D, Grubb BP, Karas BJ, et al. Exercise-induced neurocardiogenic syncope: Clinical data, pathophysiological aspects, and potential role of tilt table testing. *Europace* 2000; 2:77–82.

Olshansky B. Syncope: Overview and approach to management. In: Grubb BP, Olshansky B, eds. *Syncope: Mechanisms and Management*. Malden MA: Blackwell/Futura Publishing Co., Inc., 2005:1–47.

CHAPTER 7

Postural tachycardia syndrome and chronic fatigue syndrome

During the Civil War, doctors described seeing patients with what they termed "irritable heart syndrome" or "soldier's heart." Over the following decades, this same disorder was given many other names, including such tongue-twisters as neurocirculatory asthenia, vasoregulatory asthenia, Da Costa's syndrome, effort syndrome, postural orthostatic tachycardia syndrome, and idiopathic hypovolemia.

This condition is now commonly known as postural tachycardia syndrome (POTS). It is typically considered to be a type of neurocardiogenic syncope. Both neurocardiogenic syncope and POTS can sometimes result in a faint. Researchers now believe that there may also be considerable overlap between people with POTS and a subgroup of individuals suffering from chronic fatigue syndrome (CFS).

Common symptoms of POTS

The "postural" part of POTS refers to the fact that symptoms appear when you change your posture by standing up and disappear when you lie down. Tachycardia, of course, refers to an abnormally fast heart rate. Therefore, POTS is characterized by a very fast heart rate that occurs after you stand up. Typical symptoms of POTS include
• disabling fatigue,
• inability to perform physical activities,
• palpitations, or a rapid or throbbing sensation that feels like your heart is fluttering or beating quickly and forcefully,
• lightheadedness,
• difficulty doing exercise,
• tremulousness or involuntary trembling,
• blurred vision or "tunnel" vision,
• weakness, especially of the legs, and
• dizziness.
Other symptoms that sometimes occur in people with POTS include
• nausea,
• pain of the chest wall,
• hyperventilation, or abnormally fast breathing that causes the loss of carbon dioxide from the blood, which may result in a loss of blood pressure and fainting,

- anxiety,
- loss of concentration and memory,
- shortness of breath,
- digestive problems,
- headaches, including migraines, and
- pain or coldness of the legs, fingers, and/or ears.

Of course, if you suffer from POTS, you may also have repeated episodes in which you faint or almost faint (near-syncope).

These symptoms can profoundly affect your quality of life. People with POTS find that just eating or taking a shower may be enough to intensify their symptoms. And POTS sufferers can forget about exercise, even modest physical activity. The majority of people with POTS do not go to see a doctor when they first experience symptoms. On the average, they endure their symptoms for about a year before reporting the problem to their physician.

As with many of the underlying causes of fainting, people with POTS are often misdiagnosed as suffering from panic attacks or chronic anxiety based on the symptoms they describe. Or, most disturbing of all, when doctors do not find autonomic nervous system (ANS) failure in these patients, they may tell them that nothing is wrong with them—that it is all "in their head."

Taking a closer look at POTS

POTS is defined as the development of orthostatic symptoms as the result of an increase in heart rate of at least 30 beats per minute or a heart rate of at least 120 beats per minute occurring within the first 10 minutes of standing. This response is sometimes, but not always, associated with mild low blood pressure. When this increase in heart rate consistently results in fainting, the condition is sometimes called "POTS with syncope."

Most people with POTS are between 15 and 50 years of age, but it can occur in people younger or older than these ages. POTS is about five times more common in women than in men, and symptoms may be more likely to occur before a woman's menstrual period. Some research suggests that about half of the people with POTS had some sort of viral infection prior to the first episode during which they experienced symptoms. Some people with POTS have several days of intense symptoms, followed by periods of noticeable improvement. Other people may, on occasion, lose so much fluid (despite drinking a lot of water) that they have low blood pressure severe enough to require intravenous fluid replacement.

We currently feel that POTS is a group of related yet different disorders that produce similar symptoms. We are still trying to learn about and understand each cause of POTS, and how each cause may differ from the others.

At present we divide POTS into two major groups: primary POTS and secondary POTS. We use the term "primary POTS" to describe when the condition occurs by itself and is not associated with another condition or disorder. The term "secondary POTS" is used to describe when the condition occurs as a consequence of some other disease or condition. These individuals suffering from primary POTS can be farther subdivided into two groups: partial dysautonomic (PD) and hyperadrenergic. By far the partial PD form is the most common, accounting for close to 90% of cases. Remember when described how the normal body compensates for stress of gravity while standing? You will recall that the force of the heart's contraction and, most importantly, an increase in the vasoconstriction of blood vessels in the lower half of the body. Patients suffering from the PD form of POTS are unable to adequately cause or maintain constriction of the blood vessels in the lower half of the body while standing. The blood then pools in the large vessels of the legs and lower abdomen. The heart then receives less blood returning to the right ventricle, which in turn causes the baroreceptors in the ventricle to send messages to the parts of the brain that control heart rate and blood pressure. The brain then increases the sympathetic outflow to the heart, causing the heart contraction to increase. However, because the blood vessels are not contracting adequately, the heart rate goes excessively fast in an attempt to compensate. While this response may keep the blood pressure in the low normal range and uses tremendous amounts of energy as well. Functually it is as if the affected person is "running in place" all the time. The patient with this form of POTS can experience extreme fatigue, palpitations, inability to exercise, shortness of breath, and difficulty concentrating. At times this compensation mechanism fails and the blood pressure may fall low enough to cause a faint.

While the cause of this form of POTS is not well understood, it is generally felt that many of the patients suffer from an autoimmune disorder (the body abnormally produces antibodies against parts of itself). Many patients with this form of POTS will relate that symptoms began following a viral infection.

A second group of POTS patients either over-produce norepinephrine or have overly sensitive norepinephrine receptors. As you recall from Chapter 5, norepinephrine is a hormone that causes an increase in both heart rate and the force of the heart's contraction. A number of these patients have very high serum norepinephine levels, and this causes the heart to beat harder and faster, and often results in an initial elevation in blood pressure. Patients with this form of POTS (called hyperadrenic) also experience palpitations, as well as extreme tremor, anxiety, and sweating. As the heart rate becomes more and more rapid, it can reach a point where the ventricle does not have enough time to fill with blood prior to the contraction. This can result in a decrease in the amount of blood being pumped with each beat, which can reduce the amount of blood reaching the brain. Again, the end result will be a loss of oxygen to the brain, resulting in lightheadedness, headaches, difficulty thinking, and ultimately loss of consciousness.

A separate group of POTS patients are said to suffer from "secondary POTS". This group is composed of people with diseases that can disrupt the normal function of the ANS. For example, diabetes can damage the nerves in your body—a condition called diabetic neuropathy. When the nerves in your blood vessels are damaged, they cannot constrict the vessel wall in response to sympathetic impulses. This inability to constrict blood vessels in the lower body—legs and abdomen—means that blood flow to the heart is reduced, leading to a drop in blood pressure and the resulting symptoms. In these people, sympathetic impulses continue to work on the heart, increasing heart rate and strength of contractions. So, while heart rate speeds up, blood pressure will still be below normal, which can lead to symptoms.

Of course, a decrease in fluid volume in the body can also decrease the amount of blood returning to the heart and trigger the rapid heart rate characteristic of POTS.

Another condition that can predispose a person POTS is called "joint hypermobility syndrome." In these individuals there is a different type of collagen in parts of the body. Collagen is a substance that acts like the "glue" or "cement" of the body and serves to connect fibres together. There are multiple different types of collagen, some stronger, some weaker, some rigid, and some flexible. Patients with hypermobility syndrome have a more elastic form of collagen than usual in their skin, the ligaments of their joints, and in the walls of the blood vessels (most often veins). These individuals have soft, velvety skin, hypermobile joints, and blood vessels that stretch when subjected to a prolonged pressure load (like standing does to the lower body blood vessels). This allows blood to pool in the lower half of the body, which triggers a compensatory increase in heart rate (i.e., POTS). Sometimes serious conditions, such as cancer or multiple sclerosis, may present with POTS-like symptoms.

POTS and mitral valve prolapse

Your mitral, or bicuspid, valve is located between the left atrium and ventricle. Mitral valve prolapse is an inherited disorder in which part of the mitral valve is pushed back too far-prolapsed during the contraction of the ventricle. Since this condition prevents the mitral valve from closing properly, a small amount of blood is allowed to flow back into the left atrium when the ventricle contracts. Mitral valve prolapse is the most common abnormality in human heart valves.

When people with mitral valve prolapse have symptoms of abnormal ANS responses, they tend to be the same as in individuals with POTS. These individuals have increased levels of epinephrine and norepinephrine (see Chapter 3) and an exaggerated response of these neurotransmitters to an increase in blood volume. This results in the increased heart rate—tachycardia—that is typical of people with POTS.

POTS and chronic fatigue syndrome

You might wonder why there is a section on CFS in this chapter on POTS. The primary reason is that research has now shown that some (but not all) people with CFS also meet the criteria for POTS. It has been suggested that POTS may be an underlying cause of the symptoms of CFS in these individuals. Why is this important? There is no consistently effective treatment for CFS; however, POTS can often be successfully treated.

What is CFS?

CFS is chronic, debilitating fatigue. It most often occurs between the ages of 25 and 45, and women are twice as likely to develop it as men. It is difficult to know how many people actually have CFS—the numbers depend on how carefully the complete definition is applied. However, the Centers for Disease Control and Prevention (CDC) estimate that between two and seven people per 100,000 Americans suffer from CFS.

In order for CFS to be diagnosed, the following criteria must be met:

1. The clinically evaluated, persistent or relapsing fatigue cannot be explained by other causes. The fatigue must be new or have a definite time of onset that you can identify. Resting does not reduce the fatigue. And, the chronic fatigue results in a substantial reduction of your previous levels of occupational, social, educational, and/or personal activities.

2. You must also have four or more of the following symptoms that persist or recur during 6 or more consecutive months of illness and that did not occur before the fatigue:

(a) self-reported difficulty in short-term memory or concentration,

(b) sore throat,

(c) tender lymph nodes in the neck or armpits,

(d) muscle pain,

(e) pain that moves from one joint to another, with no redness or swelling,

(f) headaches with a new pattern or severity,

(g) sleep that does not refresh you or make you feel rested, and

(h) fatigue lasting 24 hours or more following exercise that you previously tolerated.

Potential causes of CFS

The symptoms of CFS are pretty general. As you might imagine, this makes it difficult to diagnose this disease. Diagnosis is often a case of ruling out everything else that might cause the symptoms. The National Institutes of Health (NIH) provided the following list of some common causes of chronic fatigue (see NIAID):

• underactive thyroid (hypothyroidism),

• sleep apnea (temporary stoppage of breathing while sleeping),

• narcolepsy (disorder characterized by sudden, uncontrollable, usually brief attacks of deep sleep),

• hepatitis (liver inflammation) B or C,

• alcohol and/or other substance abuse,

• severe obesity,

• side effects of medication,

• systemic lupus erythematosus ("lupus"),

• multiple sclerosis,

- cancer,
- major depression,
- eating disorders, such as anorexia or bulimia,
- schizophrenia,
- dementia, and
- manic-depressive (bipolar) disorder.

If the doctor cannot identify one of these causes or find another underlying cause for the chronic fatigue being experienced, CFS is the diagnosis that is left. It is important for people with CFS to be evaluated for POTS, even in the absence of fainting. This is usually done using the tilt-table test, which will be discussed in Chapter 10. If POTS is found to be the underlying cause of the CFS, the symptoms may be reversible with therapies used to treat POTS. These treatments will be covered in Chapter 11.

Looking forward . . .

Chapter 8 contains information about some miscellaneous causes of fainting. A few of them may actually seem a little odd, but all of them can be serious if they lead to fall-related injuries.

References

Gazit Y, Nahir M, Grahame R, et al. Dysautonomia in the joint hypermobility syndrome. *American Journal of Medicine* 2003;115:33–40.

Grubb BP. Idiopathic postural orthostatic tachycardia: A variant of neurocardiogenic syncope? In: Raviele A, ed. *Cardiac Arrhythmias 1999*. Milan: Springer-Verlag, 2000: 430–436.

Grubb BP, Calkins H, Rowe PC. Postural tachycardia, orthostatic intolerance, and the chronic fatigue syndrome. In: Grubb BP, Olshansky B, eds. *Syncope: Mechanisms and Management*. Malden, MA: Blackwell/Futura Press, 2005: 225–244.

Grubb BP, Kanjwal Y, Kosinski D. The postural tachycardia syndrome: A concise guide to diagnosis and management. *Journal of Cardiac Electrophysiology* 2006;17:108–112.

Low PA, Opfer-Gehrking TL, Textor SC, et al. Comparison of the postural tachycardia syndrome (POTS) with orthostatic hypotension due to autonomic failure. *Journal of the Autonomic Nervous System* 1994;50:181–188.

Low PA, Opfer-Gehrking TL, Textor SC, et al. Postural tachycardia syndrome (POTS). *Neurology* 1995;45(suppl 5):519–525.

Low PA, Schondorf R, Novak V, et al. Postural tachycardia syndrome. In: Low PA, ed. *Clinical Autonomic Disorders*, 2nd edition. Philadelphia: Lippincott-Raven Publishers, 1977: 681–697.

NIAID (National Institute of Allergy and Infectious Diseases). Chronic fatigue syndrome. www.niaid.nih.gov/publications/cfs/complete.htm.

Sandroni P, Opfer-Gehrking TL, McPhee BR, et al. Postural tachycardia syndrome: Clinical features and follow-up study. *Mayo Clinic Proceedings* 1999;74:1106–1110.

Steward JM, Gewitz MA, Weldon A, et al. Orthostatic intolerance in adolescent chronic fatigue syndrome. *Pediatrics* 1999;103:116–121.

Other possible causes of fainting

Some conditions or diseases have a complete list of causes that is generally agreed upon by almost everyone. Unfortunately, this is not the case with the many and varied underlying causes of fainting. In fact, it would be a rare occurrence to find any two experts who would approach this information in exactly the same way. The main purpose of this book, however, is not to develop yet another complicated list of causes for fainting. It is meant to provide the most useful information to you, the reader—the person who may be experiencing faints. This chapter is actually a sort of "grab bag" of various other causes of fainting.

You have probably already noticed that there is considerable overlap in many of the conditions that can cause fainting. This will become even more obvious in this chapter since some of the underlying causes of fainting discussed here may have already been mentioned in earlier chapters.

Other common causes of fainting

First, it is important to keep in mind that no underlying cause can be identified in a large proportion of people who faint. Out of the causes that are identified, neurocardiogenic syncope appears to be the most common. Next is orthostatic hypotension, which itself has many underlying causes, including failure of the autonomic nervous system (ANS), drugs, reduced blood volume, or a combination of factors.

Postprandial hypotension

Postprandial hypotension as a cause of fainting was touched on in Chapters 5 and 6. Postprandial hypotension is often defined as a fall in systolic blood pressure of 20 mm Hg or more within 2 hours of starting a meal. This condition is present to some degree in many very elderly people.

Although blood pools in the abdomen during the digestion of food, this pooling alone does not appear to lead to symptomatic low blood pressure. Healthy people typically have some decrease in blood pressure as the result of eating. However, eating also stimulates the sympathetic nervous system, which normally speeds up heart rate and increases the constriction of blood vessels, both of which help maintain blood pressure. In fact, most people continue to have an adequate supply of blood being returned to and subsequently pumped out of the heart after eating.

Researchers now believe that postprandial hypotension is controlled by a factor in the lower digestive tract—the gut—which causes the dilation of blood vessels. This factor is released in response to the consumption of food. Carbohydrates—sugars and starches—are more likely to cause postprandial hypotension.

People with postprandial hypotension typically experience dizziness or faint after eating. Fainting can cause falls, of course, which may result in injuries and lead to disability, especially in older people. Other symptoms may include blurred vision, weakness, lightheadedness, vague feelings of discomfort (malaise), disturbed speech, nausea, chest pain (when blood pressure is low), or transient ischemic attacks—temporary blockage in the brain's blood supply, sometimes called a "mini-stroke."

Sick sinus syndrome

The atrioventricular (AV) node located in the wall of the right atrium is also called the sinus node. As was discussed in Chapter 4, the sinus node is your heart's internal "pacemaker," initiating each separate heartbeat and setting the pace for the heart. Its proper functioning is key to the heart's independent conduction (electrical) system.

Both bradyarrhythmia (irregular slow heart rate) and tachyarrhythmia (irregular fast heart rate) can cause the symptoms that precede a faint. These abnormal heart rates can result from any number of malfunctions of the sinus node. You may sometimes hear these malfunctions grouped together under the general terms "sinoatrial disease" or "sick sinus syndrome." Sick sinus syndrome is especially common in older individuals.

People with sick sinus syndrome most often report dizziness, lightheadedness, shortness of breath, palpitations, fatigue, sluggishness, lack of interest in their surroundings, fainting, and even dementia (deterioration of mental faculties, such as concentration, memory, and judgment). When sick sinus syndrome results in a slowed heartbeat, or bradycardia, it may cause symptoms—especially during physical activity—but rarely leads to an outright faint.

At times, sick sinus syndrome may manifest itself as periods of bradycardia alternating with very rapid, uncoordinated contractions of the atria (atrial fibrillation). In this case, the symptoms may be the result of the bradycardia, the atrial fibrillation (or another form of tachycardia), or both. Another possible cause of dizziness and fainting in people with sick sinus syndrome is the occurrence of a long pause in heartbeat following an episode of rapid heart rate.

Sinus node function can also be affected by a number of medications. These include some antiarrhythmic drugs (to control irregular heartbeat), antihypertensive drugs (to control high blood pressure), beta-adrenergic blocking drugs (to reduce heart rate and the force of heart contractions), and calcium channel blockers (to relax heart muscle and slow heart rate).

AV block

AV block refers to a blocking of the normal activity of the AV node (see Chapter 4). This node located in the wall that separates the two atria has the important job of slowing down nerve impulses before sending them to the ventricles and causing them to contract. This very brief pause allows the atria to finish emptying the blood they are holding into the ventricles.

When the AV node slows down the conduction of the nerve impulses for a longer period than normal, it is known as first-degree AV block. If the AV node sometimes fails to pass on nerve impulses at all, it is second-degree AV block. Third-degree AV block refers to complete failure of the AV node to pass on any nerve impulses.

There are several potential causes of AV block. It can result from age-related changes to the heart's conduction system, heart attack, chronic heart disease in which there is decreased blood flow to the arteries of the heart, certain drugs, inflammatory diseases, and tumors, among other causes.

Ventricular tachycardia

Ventricular tachycardia (VT) refers to an abnormally rapid contraction of the ventricles. It is defined as three or more consecutive ventricular premature beats. VT can be nonsustained, which means that it lasts less than 30 seconds, or it can be sustained. Because ventricles contracting too quickly are not able to pump the normal amount of blood with each beat, the blood flow to the brain may be insufficient, leading to a faint.

VT often results in palpitations, dizziness, lightheadedness, and a drop in blood pressure that causes fainting. VT is a common complication of heart attack and several other forms of heart abnormalities or diseases. If not controlled, VT can sometimes be fatal.

Situational syncope

Situational syncope is a very general term that refers to fainting in response to a particular situation. Many of these situations result in a faint because they somehow cause an increase in pressure inside the chest. Remember that anything that increases the pressure inside your chest may potentially decrease the amount of blood able to pass through that area on its way to your heart. When the ANS is not able to compensate for this increase in internal chest pressure, there can be a reduction in blood being pumped to your brain, resulting in a faint.

Situational syncope includes a number of varied causes, some of which may seem a bit unusual or even bizarre. For example, some people faint when they suddenly get up from a hot tub or jacuzzi. In this instance, the blood vessels in their lower body have expanded in response to the heat. When they stand, they just are not able to compensate for the blood pooling in the enlarged blood vessels.

Have you ever seen children who hold their breath until they faint? This is another type of situational syncope. As a child, were you ever warned not to drink a cold beverage when you were very hot? This advice may originally have been based on the fact that people with "swallow syncope" may experience a drop in blood pressure and lowered heart rate in response to a cold drink. As you know by now, this response can lead to fainting. Some people increase the pressure within their chest to the point of fainting when they play a trumpet, urinate, pass stool, cough, or even sneeze.

Sexual activity is associated with stimulation of sympathetic responses. In some individuals, this type of activity can actually cause them to faint. A number of individuals suffering from a blockage of an artery in the lung by a blood clot (pulmonary embolism) may report fainting as a symptom when visiting the doctor.

Some athletes have fainting episodes either during vigorous activity, moderate activity, or even at rest. Researchers have noted that a sizeable proportion of athletes who suffer sudden death had a history of fainting. This makes it especially important to identify and, when possible, treat the underlying cause of this problem in these individuals.

Some individuals with pacemakers experience episodes of fainting. Doctors used to believe that this was a result of a malfunctioning pacemaker. However, recent research indicates that these people most likely faint as the result of neurocardiogenic syncope.

One of the rarer causes of fainting is a type of neurocardiogenic syncope associated with, of all things, hair grooming. Hair-grooming syncope seizures generally occur in young women who experience nausea, lightheadedness, sweating, and visual disturbances prior to fainting. How does this happen? Researchers think that the pulling of the hair or stimulation of the scalp has an effect on a particular nerve in the head that triggers the fainting response.

Fainting due to drugs

As you already know, fainting can be a side effect of a number of drugs in some people. The main culprits among prescription drugs are those used to treat high blood pressure. Drugs designed to lower heart rate or promote vasodilation make it harder for the body to compensate for changes in blood volume and blood pressure. This can lead to a decreased blood flow to the brain and fainting. Table 5-4 lists the most common types of drugs that cause orthostatic hypotension, which can lead to fainting.

In addition, alcohol can cause an irregular heart rate. This condition is sometimes called the "holiday heart" syndrome because it is associated with the overindulgence in alcohol that seems to be characteristic of some holidays. Cocaine may also cause fainting secondary to the irregular heartbeat stemming from other conditions.

More miscellaneous causes of fainting

A relatively few people faint due to low blood sugar levels (hypoglycemia), hyperventilation (abnormally fast breathing that causes the loss of carbon dioxide from the blood), or low levels of oxygen in the blood or body tissues (hypoxia). At times having too much or too little potassium, calcium, or magnesium in the blood can cause a person to faint.

In addition, some disorders of the endocrine system can potentially lead to a faint. For example, low activity of the adrenal gland, such as in Addison's disease, can result in orthostatic hypotension and fainting.

Looking forward . . .

The next chapter applies the information on underlying causes of fainting discussed in Chapters 5 through 8 specifically to children and adolescents and to older individuals.

References

Benditt DG, Sutton R. Bradyarrhythmias as a cause of syncope. In: Grubb BP, Olshansky B, eds. *Syncope: Mechanisms and Management*. Malden, MA: Blackwell/Futura Publishing Co., Inc., 2005: 92–120.

Hedrich O, Link M, Homoud M, et al. Syncope in the athlete. In: Grubb BP, Olshansky B, eds. *Syncope: Mechanisms and Management*. Malden, MA: Blackwell/Futura Publishing Co., Inc., 2006: 287–300.

Jansen RWMM, Lipsitz LA. Postprandial hypotension: Epidemiology, pathophysiology, and clinical management. *Annals of Internal Medicine* 1995; 122: 286–295.

Kosinski DJ, Grubb BP. Miscellaneous causes of syncope. In: Grubb BP, Olshansky B, eds. *Syncope: Mechanisms and Management*. Malden, MA: Blackwell/Futura Publishing Co., Inc., 2005: 267–272.

Pelosi F, Morady F. Tachyarrhythmias as a cause of syncope. In: Grubb BP, Olshansky B, eds. *Syncope: Mechanisms and Management*. Malden, MA: Blackwell Futura Publishing Co., Inc., 2005: 121–125.

CHAPTER 9

Fainting in children and adolescents and in older people

This chapter explores the role of fainting at two ends of the age spectrum—in children and adolescents and in older people. Although these two age groups share many causes of fainting with people in their middle years, they also have some interesting differences.

Fainting in children and adolescents

It might surprise you to know that fainting is fairly common in children and adolescents. In fact, an estimated 15–50% of children will have had at least one fainting episode by the time they become adults (Prodinger and Reisdorff, 1998).

Common causes of fainting in children and adolescents

One way to look at the causes of fainting in young people is to divide them into broad classifications. First, there are causes related to alterations in the control of heart rate and blood pressure by the autonomic nervous system (ANS) (see Chapter 3). Second, there are causes associated with the heart itself. Third, there is a sort of "catchall" that basically includes everything else.

Fainting and the ANS

There are three primary conditions that can result in fainting due to temporary changes in the control of heart rate and blood pressure by the ANS. This category includes neurocardiogenic syncope (see Chapter 6), orthostatic hypotension (see Chapter 5), and cerebral vasoconstriction, or the abnormal constriction of blood vessels in the brain.

Neurocardiogenic syncope

Neurocardiogenic syncope is the most common cause of fainting in otherwise healthy children and adolescents. As with adults, a sudden fall in blood pressure first causes the heart rate to speedup and then to slow. The symptoms that typically occur before the actual loss of consciousness include lightheadedness, dizziness, sweating and a sensation of warmth, nausea, pallor, and a slow visual loss. When children begin to experience these symptoms, they tend to panic. Their anxiety often causes them to hyperventilate.

What can cause neurocardiogenic syncope in a youngster? These episodes are often triggered by something in the environment. Anxiety or pain can lead to fainting. Drawing a blood sample or even just the sight of blood may result in neurocardiogenic syncope in some children. At times, all it may take is seeing a needle. In other cases, children may just be going about their routine activities—playing, walking, coughing, urinating, passing stool, or crying—when they suddenly become sweaty and pale and faint. This, of course, is very frightening, both for the youngsters and their parents, siblings, and other people close to them.

Adolescents often have had a period of rapid growth before they begin to experience symptoms of neurocardiogenic syncope. It appears that fainting episodes are more likely to occur in young women before their menstrual periods. Some research indicates that fainting episodes are also more common in adolescents who crash diet, losing a large amount of weight in a relatively short period of time.

Orthostatic hypotension

What occurs in children and adolescents with orthostatic hypotension is the same as in adults. There is a pooling of blood in the lower body upon standing. Normally, the ANS would trigger a reflex-controlled increase in heart rate and force of contraction and a constriction of blood vessels—all of which would help increase blood pressure. In orthostatic hypotension, however, the ANS fails to compensate for the blood pooling, which can lead to insufficient blood reaching the brain and, ultimately, fainting.

Compared with neurocardiogenic syncope, orthostatic hypotension usually has fewer warning symptoms. Doctors may suspect it when the faint follows a change in position. There typically is no slowing of heartbeat or increase in sweating in children and adolescents who faint due to orthostatic hypotension.

Cerebral syncope

Recently, researchers have found that a few children and adolescents may faint as the result of what is called cerebral syncope. In these cases, the mechanism appears to be a limitation in blood flow to the brain due to a constriction of the blood vessels in the brain itself. These episodes are often associated with migraines. Patients frequently report a sudden fainting spell that occurs with little warning after which they wake up with a migraine headache.

Fainting and the heart

Heart-related causes for fainting are often called cardiac or cardiovascular syncope. These terms refer to fainting due to changes in blood flow or to alterations in normal heart rhythm.

Lack of oxygen

Sometimes children experience a fall in the level of oxygen in their blood. Have you ever seen children go from crying to taking quick, deep breaths? As the crying forces air out of their lungs, they experience an increase in pressure in their chest. This reduces the amount of blood reaching the lungs to pick up needed oxygen. If the level of oxygen in the blood drops low enough, the youngster will lose consciousness.

The best way to try to head off this type of faint is to calm the children. Then, have them squat and bring their knees to their chest. This will increase the constriction of blood vessels in the lower body, thereby helping normalize blood flow to the lungs.

Obstructed blood flow

Any condition that obstructs blood flow out of the heart reduces cardiac output, which, as you recall, is the amount of blood your left ventricle ejects into the aorta during systole in a minute (see Chapter 4). Any narrowing or constriction of the aortic valve or the area around it can lead to obstructed blood flow. The aortic valve controls blood flow from the left ventricle into the aorta. A number of conditions can obstruct the flow of blood to the lungs (pulmonary embolism), heart (heart attack), or brain (stroke). All of these situations can sometimes result in a fainting episode.

Abnormal heart rhythms

In most cases, a child or adolescent whose heart is free of structural abnormalities will not have rhythm disturbances severe enough to cause a faint. However, children may experience a number of inherited (congenital) or acquired irregularities in heart rhythm that can lead to fainting. Many of these potential causes are discussed in Chapter 8. In children, the most common underlying cause of irregular heartbeat that leads to fainting is congenital heart disease. The abnormal rhythm may actually occur after a congenital defect has been corrected. Sometimes emotion or exercise causes fainting in a youngster with a structurally normal heart. In these cases, the doctor may want to consider a type of syncope resulting from ventricular tachycardia—rapid contraction of the ventricles. This condition is of special importance because it may have a high mortality rate if not treated, usually with beta-blocking drugs.

"Catchall" category

There are several other causes of fainting in children and adolescents that do not fall into the preceding categories. They include such causes as hysteric syncope, epilepsy, hyperventilation, and fainting due to drug use.

Hysteric syncope

Hysteric syncope is an important cause of fainting in children and especially in adolescents. Individuals with hysteric syncope often faint several times in a day and may be unconscious for a long period, some times as long as an hour. Hysteric syncope differs from most other causes of fainting in that these individuals have a normal heart rate and blood pressure and do not regain consciousness when they lie flat. People with hysteric syncope often seem to be unconcerned with their fainting problem.

Hysteric syncope is sometimes due to what is called a conversion disorder, which consists of symptoms that suggest a nervous system problem but are caused by psychological factors. In this instance, the conversion disorder is often the result of past physical or sexual abuse.

Epilepsy

Seizures, such as are characteristic of epilepsy, are not actually a common cause of syncope. When fainting does occur with a seizure, there is typically incontinence (lack of bladder and bowel control), tonic-clonic movements (both prolonged contractions and alternating contraction and relaxation of muscles), and loss of consciousness for a prolonged period. The seizure is often so dramatic that onlookers describe the person as being "thrown to the ground," which can result in serious injuries to the face and head. This type of seizure occurs most often in children between the ages of 2 and 8, and it rarely occurs in adolescents.

Hyperventilation

In hyperventilation, people breathe more rapidly and deeply than usual. Strange as it sounds, this causes them to feel like they cannot get enough air. They then become anxious, panicky, and desperate—gasping for breath.

Hyperventilation causes too much oxygen to be inhaled and higher than normal amounts of carbon dioxide to be exhaled. This throws the concentrations of these two gases in the blood out of balance. Too little carbon dioxide in the blood reduces the stimulation of chemoreceptors, which means that the nervous system is not able to send the impulses that would normalize breathing. The result is that the blood supply to the brain is further reduced, potentially leading to a faint. These episodes can last up to half an hour.

The best way to treat hyperventilation is to try to calm these individuals, encouraging them to breathe more normally. Having them temporarily hold their breath may help. One old remedy is to have the person breathe into a paper bag. This causes rebreathing of air that has been exhaled from the lungs, which is higher in carbon dioxide. If someone who is hyperventilating faints, the ANS typically takes over and normalizes breathing. Sometimes biofeedback is helpful in controlling hyperventilation.

Drug use

There are instances in which someone will faint due to using—or, as is often the case, misusing—drugs. It is unfortunate, but this problem is all too common in young people. These individuals are often indifferent to the dangers associated with their fainting episodes. They may be openly hostile to the doctor and typically volunteer little or no information that would help in a diagnosis of their problem.

Fainting in older people

If fainting is such an important cause of disability in older people, why would this topic be saved until last? For one thing, just about everything that has been discussed in the chapters on orthostatic hypotension, neurocardiogenic syncope, postural tachycardia syndrome, and the other common causes of fainting is also true for older people. But there are several reasons why older individuals may be more vulnerable to the underlying causes for fainting than are younger people.

Special concerns in older individuals

First, older people are more likely to suffer from chronic medical problems that can increase their chances of fainting. Diabetes, congestive heart failure, coronary artery disease, and cerebrovascular disease, for example, occur more often in this population. Second, older individuals are more likely to be using one or more medications that may cause fainting. It is not unusual for an older person to be taking sedatives, diuretics, vasodilators, and/or beta-blocking drugs, all of which may contribute to fainting. Third, there is the aging process itself. Older people are more likely to have physical changes that may limit the amount of blood able to reach the brain.

You may recall from Chapter 2 that fainting accounts for 3% of all visits to the emergency room and up to 6% of all hospital admissions. However, the startling fact is that 80% of these people are over age 65. Serious injury and even death stemming from a fainting episode is much more common in older individuals.

One of the major concerns with fainting is the potential injury that may be sustained during the fall that often results from a faint. Of course, there are a number of risk factors for falls in older people. External causes, such as slipping on a loose throw rug or slippery floor, account for about half the falls in the elderly. Orthostatic intolerance is one of the underlying causes for the remaining 50% of falls. Each year, approximately 30% of people over age 65 and 50% of those over 85 who are living on their own experience a fall (Steinweg, 1997). People in nursing homes fare even worse. Up to half of the residents of nursing homes fall each year, and more than 40% of them fall more than once.

What is the actual impact of these falls on health? From 30% to 50% of falls result in minor injuries that do not need medical attention and thus are not reflected in the treatment statistics. In 1996, there were 21,712,000 visits to a medical office or facility for a fall (NCHS, 1996, Table 9). Falls typically result in injuries such as fractured bones, superficial injuries, open wounds and lacerations, sprains and strains, and other injuries. In 1995, falls accounted for 23% of injury deaths in people age 65 and older and 34% in people 85 and older. Because of the ways doctors code certain causes of death, these estimates are most likely low (NCHS, 1997).

Common causes of fainting in older people

There are a number of common causes of fainting in older individuals. By now, they should be at least somewhat familiar to you.

Postprandial hypotension

Postprandial hypotension—a drop in blood pressure when you stand up after eating—is one of the most common causes of fainting in the older population. In older individuals, postprandial hypotension appears to be the result of an inability of the sympathetic nervous system to compensate for the blood that pools around the digestive organs after a meal.

Sometimes the symptoms of postprandial hypotension are subtle in older people, who may attribute the slight dizziness or weakness they experience when standing after eating to something else, even aging itself. After all, the symptoms may not appear until more than an hour after the meal. However, fainting, falling, and sustaining potentially serious injuries are very real dangers in this age group.

Orthostatic hypotension

There is an increased prevalence of orthostatic hypotension in older people. In one study, 347 randomly picked people, age 56 or older, were evaluated for orthostatic hypotension. In this group, 28% of the people had a drop in systolic blood pressure of at least 20 mm Hg after standing for 3 minutes (Raiha et al., 1995). It has been estimated that as many as 30% of the people over age 65 living outside extended-care nursing facilities have orthostatic hypotension. In another study, researchers found that more than half of frail people, age 60 and older, who were living in a nursing home, experienced orthostatic hypotension, especially in the morning (Ooi et al., 1997).

Many older people have fairly broad swings in blood pressure throughout the day without experiencing symptoms. However, they may faint when a number of factors combine to reduce the supply of blood to the brain.

Research has shown that the degree of fall in blood pressure that is defined as orthostatic hypotension is more common when the initial blood pressure is high-hypertension. The fact that older people are more likely to have high blood pressure makes them also at higher risk of orthostatic hypotension. In addition, as you have seen in the section on medications, many of the drugs that can cause orthostatic hypotension are used to treat high blood pressure. Older people also tend to have a higher systolic blood pressure when lying down—supine hypertension. This encourages a greater relative drop in blood pressure upon standing.

A number of other changes associated with aging can also increase the odds of developing orthostatic hypotension. Older people may have baroreceptors that are less sensitive to changes in blood pressure. This means that the cardiovascular center in the brain does not consistently receive the signal to increase sympathetic impulses, which increase heart rate and constrict blood vessels—two mechanisms for increasing blood pressure.

In an older person, the heart is slower to respond to changes in blood pressure. There is also an age-related decline in the responses of the ANS. In addition, older individuals are more likely to have a disorder of the ANS, which helps regulate blood pressure. This may decrease the ability of blood vessels to constrict, making it less likely that an older person can compensate adequately when low blood pressure occurs upon standing.

The aging kidney often loses sodium, which increases urination and decreases blood volume. Older people typically have lower levels of renin, angiotensin, and aldosterone, and these levels do not rise as much as in younger people upon standing. Older individuals are more likely to have one or more of the diseases or conditions that are secondary causes of neurocardiogenic orthostatic hypotension (see Chapter 5). Sometimes orthostatic hypotension may result from a poor nutritional state. For example, anemia or a low level of potassium in the blood (hypokalemia) can both contribute to orthostatic hypotension.

Orthostatic hypotension is of special concern in older individuals. The falls that can result from dizziness or fainting may potentially cause physical injuries serious enough to result in permanent disability or even death in this age group.

Heart-related faints

Some studies suggest that 21–34% of the fainting episodes in older people are due to some type of heart-related cause. Following are the primary heart-related causes of fainting in this age group:
• Various types of irregular heartbeats, or arrhythmias (see Chapter 8).
• Sick sinus syndrome, which is a malfunction of the sinus node, the heart's internal pacemaker (see Chapter 8).
• Aortic stenosis, which is a narrowing of the valve through which blood is pumped out of the left ventricle (the heart's main pumping chamber) and into the aorta (the main artery of the body).
• Heart attack, which is the result of blocking the flow of blood in an artery in the heart muscle itself.
• Heart block (AV block), which refers to a situation in which electrical impulses pass through the AV node and bundle of His (see Chapter 4) either very slowly, only some of the time, or not at all.

Aortic stenosis is an especially important heart-related cause for fainting in older people. Once people reach age 85, the vast majority of them have at least some hardening of the aortic valve. Although symptoms due to aortic stenosis typically occur with exercise, they can also be caused by a hot bath or a vasodilator medication, that is, one that enlarges the blood vessels in the body.

Another underlying cause of fainting that is often overlooked is pulmonary embolism. Pulmonary embolism results from a piece of a blood clot formed somewhere else in the body traveling through the heart and blocking an artery in the lungs. The clots that cause a pulmonary embolism often come from a deep vein thrombosis, that is, a blood clot that is formed in the veins located deep in the legs or groin areas of the body. One of the risk factors for deep vein thrombosis is a slowed blood flow back to the heart.

Disorders of the nervous system

As you get older, you are more likely to develop a malfunction of the ANS. For example, older individuals may have problems of the ANS associated with other diseases, including

- Parkinson's disease,
- chronic strokes,
- multiple system atrophy (Shy-Drager syndrome),
- Huntington's disease,
- Guillain-Barré syndrome,
- pure autonomic failure (Bradbury-Eggleston syndrome),
- diabetes mellitus,
- tabes dorsalis,
- amyloidosis,
- porphyria,
- alcoholism,
- specific spinal cord problems, and
- disorders of the peripheral nerves.

ANS problems

How can you tell if you have problems with your ANS? One way is to be aware of the symptoms so that you can be sure to report them to your doctor. The most common symptoms associated with a malfunction of the ANS include

- postural, or orthostatic, hypotension,
- fainting,
- fatigue,
- reduced sweating,
- constipation,
- loss of urinary control or inability to empty the bladder,
- disturbances in vision, and
- erectile dysfunction and impotence in men.

Transient ischemic attacks

If you think about it, fainting has a lot in common with a transient ischemic attack (TIA). A TIA, which is sometimes referred to as a "mini-stroke," is a temporary blockage of the blood supply to the brain. It is a short-term condition, usually lasting 10 minutes or less. A TIA typically causes dizziness, blurred vision, numbness on one side of the body, and other symptoms associated with a stroke. The blockage is usually caused by a blood clot and may be a sign of cerebrovascular disease, that is, some disease process involving the blood vessels of the brain. Fainting can be the result of cerebrovascular disease, but this is not a common cause.

It is important to discover whether a TIA or neurocardiogenic syncope is causing the symptoms. If the symptoms are caused by TIAs, they may warn you that you are at increased risk of having a stroke. When symptoms are due to neurocardiogenic syncope, however, they can typically be improved by the therapies discussed in Chapter 11.

Reflex mechanisms

You are probably familiar with the term "reflex." It refers to an involuntary reaction to a stimulus. Think of the old knee-jerk reaction when the doctor tapped you on the knee with the rubber hammer. Reflex mechanisms automatically occur in a given situation but, when they somehow go wrong, they can lead to fainting.

Carotid sinus hypersensitivity

About 10% of older people have what is called carotid sinus hypersensitivity. Think back to Chapter 4 wherein you learned that some of the baroreceptors that detect an increase in blood pressure are found in the neck. More specifically, these pressure receptors are located in the carotid sinus, an enlarged area of the common carotid artery, which carries blood from the heart to the brain. In addition to baroreceptors, the carotid sinus also contains chemoreceptors (see Chapter 4), making it very important in the reflex (automatic) control of heart rate, blood pressure, and the degree of dilation of your blood vessels.

People with carotid sinus hypersensitivity have a greater than normal response to pressure on the baroreceptors in the carotid sinus. There are three basic responses to these baroreceptors. One type of response results in bradycardia—slowing of your heartbeat—or even a block of the AV node. A second possible response does not slow the heartbeat but does reduce the constriction of blood vessels, which results in lower blood pressure. The third type of response basically combines the first two—there is a slowing of the heartbeat plus enlargement of blood vessels.

Carotid sinus hypersensitivity appears to be more common in men who have high blood pressure or coronary heart disease. Risk of carotid sinus hypersensitivity is also greater in people taking digitalis (for congestive heart failure and certain other heart problems), methyldopa (for high blood pressure), or beta-blocking drugs (for high blood pressure and certain other heart problems).

Increased pressure in the chest

In Chapter 8, you read about different types of situations that can cause a faint. Fainting in response to a temporary reduction of blood flow to the heart due to increased pressure in the chest is considered a type of reflex syncope, or faint. As you may recall, internal chest pressure can be increased by coughing, sneezing, or straining when you urinate or pass stool, all of which are considered reflex activities in this context. Blood flow through the chest area can also be temporarily reduced when you strain to lift heavy weights.

Neurocardiogenic syncope

Chapter 6 covered neurocardiogenic syncope in some detail. However, it is important to note that this condition is often also grouped under the heading of a reflex mechanism. When blood pools in your lower body upon standing, the supply of blood to your heart is reduced. Your ventricles contract harder in an effort to compensate for the decrease in blood flow. The baroreceptors in the ventricles typically respond to the pressure of excess blood in the ventricle, signaling an increase in heart rate and constriction of your blood vessels to lower blood pressure. This is the normal reflex mechanism to guard against blood pressure that is too high.

As you may recall, in certain people, the baroreceptors mistake the harder contraction of the ventricle wall for pressure from blood inside the ventricle. In this instance, the baroreceptors send messages that indicate high blood pressure instead of identifying a decrease in blood flow. Therefore, the reflex mechanism has misfired and triggered a response that is exactly opposite of what is needed. The resulting slower heartbeat and expanded blood vessels further lower blood pressure, compounding and prolonging the problem.

Although neurocardiogenic syncope does occur in older people, it is considered more common in younger individuals as a cause of fainting. When neurocardiogenic syncope does occur in elderly individuals, it has less typical symptoms and is sometimes mistaken for a TIA.

Diseases of the endocrine system

Your endocrine system includes the pituitary, thyroid, parathyroid, adrenal, pineal, and thymus glands. In addition, there are several organs in the body that contain some endocrine tissues. They include the pancreas, hypothalamus, ovaries, testes, kidneys, stomach, liver, small intestine, skin, heart, and placenta (during pregnancy). What does it mean for a tissue to have endocrine function? Endocrine glands and tissues are capable of secreting hormones, which have the job of altering the physiological activity of other tissues in the body.

Your endocrine system works together with your nervous system to coordinate the functions of all the systems in your body. As was discussed in Chapter 3, your nervous system uses substances called neurotransmitters to carry nerve impulses. Your endocrine glands, on the other hand, secrete hormones that have many activities in the body, including regulating the contraction of heart muscle and controlling fluid balance.

Diabetes is considered an endocrine disease since it is concerned with the hormone insulin, which is produced by special cells in the pancreas gland. There are a number of ways diabetes might cause fainting, including damage to the nerves that control the contraction of blood vessels.

Other causes of orthostatic hypotension and fainting associated with endocrine disorders include Addison's disease, chronic suppression of the adrenal glands from the use of steroids, and underactive pituitary gland (hypopituitarism). All of these conditions can cause a low blood volume and blood sugar, both of which can cause fainting. Diabetes insipidus, which was previously mentioned in Chapter 5, can cause fluid loss and, potentially, fainting.

Looking forward . . .

In Chapter 10, you will learn how the underlying causes of fainting are identified. Accurate diagnosis is essential since it typically determines the most appropriate and potentially successful treatment.

References

Grubb BP, Friedman R. Syncope in the child and adolescent. In: Grubb BP, Olshansky B, eds. *Syncope: Mechanisms and Management*. Malden, MA: Blackwell/Futura Publishing Co., Inc., 2005: 305–316.

Grubb BP, Samoil D, Temesy-Armos P, et al. Episodic periods of neurally mediated hypotension and bradycardia mimicking transient ischemic attacks in the elderly: Identification with head-up tilt-table testing. *Cardiology in the Elderly* 1993; 1:221–225.

Kapoor W, Snustad D, Peterson J, et al. Syncope in the elderly. *American Journal of Medicine* 1986; 80:419–428.

Lipsitz LA, Grubb BP. Syncope in the elderly. In: Grubb BP, Olshansky B, eds. *Syncope: Mechanisms and Management*. Malden, MA: Blackwell/ Futura Publishing Co., Inc., 2005:301–314.

Masuo K, Mikami H, Ogihara T, et al. Changes in frequency of orthostatic hypotension in elderly hypertensive patients under medications. *American Journal of Hypertension* 1996; 9:263–268.

NCHS (National Center for Health Statistics). Health, United States, 1996–1997, and Injury Chartbook. Hyattsville, MD: 1997.

NCHS (National Center for Health Statistics). Table 9. Number, percent distribution, and annual rate of injury-related ambulatory care visits, according to intent, mechanism, and ambulatory care setting: United States, 1996. www.cdc.gov/nchswww/data/sr13_134.pdf. Accessed April 25, 2000.

Ooi WL, Barrett S, Hossain M, et al. Patterns of orthostatic blood pressure change and their clinical correlates in a frail, elderly population. *Journal of the American Medical Association* (JAMA) 1997; 277:1299–1304.

Prodinger RJ, Reisdorff EJ. Syncope in children. *Emergency Medical Clinics of North America* 1998; 16(3):617–626.

Raiha I, Luutonen S, Piha J, et al. Prevalence, predisposing factors, and prognostic importance of postural hypotension. *Archives of Internal Medicine* 1995; 155:930–935.

Steinweg KK. The changing approach to falls in the elderly. *American Family Physician* 1997; 56:1815–1823.

CHAPTER 10

Diagnosing the underlying causes of fainting

At this point, you have become familiar with more causes of fainting than you probably ever knew existed. Now comes the tricky part. How is your doctor going to be able to identify which of the many possible underlying causes is actually responsible for your fainting? This can be a real diagnostic challenge!

Doctors who are good detectives may be able to help you avoid some unnecessary and expensive tests. The process of diagnosing the underlying cause for your faint and the other symptoms associated with it always starts with a careful history and physical examination.

Your history

Keep in mind that in order to be useful, a history must be a collaborative effort. You are responsible for giving your doctor all the basic relevant information. Next, your doctor helps make sure your history is complete by careful questioning. However, it is vital that you volunteer information—do not make the mistake of waiting for your doctor to dig out every detail. Remember that if you do not provide your doctor with all of the essential facts needed to help diagnose the underlying cause of your fainting, you are the one who loses!

Following are some questions to help you to identify the type of information your doctor will need to know:
- What is your age?
- What are your major symptoms?
- How long have you been experiencing symptoms and/or your fainting problem?
- How often do you faint?
- Do the symptoms occur when you are doing something specific, feeling any particular way, or at any particular time of day? For example, are you more likely to experience symptoms following a meal, when the weather or other environment is hot, after standing a long time in one spot, following exercise, or when you are stressed, tense, or upset?
- Exactly what happens when you faint? How long are you unconscious?
- Do you typically have symptoms just before you faint? What about any symptoms after you regain consciousness? Describe these symptoms.
- Can you connect the beginning—the onset—of your symptoms with any other event, for example, an infection of some sort?
- How long you can stand before you begin to have symptoms?

- How much have the symptoms limited your daily activities?
- Have you found any activity or remedy that relieves the symptoms?
- Are you being treated for any illness? (It is especially important to mention any heart or blood vessel disease.)
- What medications are you taking? (Be sure to list the dosage and how often you take each one.) This should also include all over-the-counter medications and other products such as vitamins, supplements, herbs, etc., that you take.
- Do you have a family history of fainting? What illnesses or conditions are common in your family? Have there been any cases of sudden death in your family?

As you can see, these questions take some thought in order to answer them completely and accurately. How many times have you been halfway home from a medical appointment before you thought of some fact you meant to tell your doctor or a question that you intended to ask? It is a smart idea to jot down the details of what has been happening *before* you keep your medical appointment. It is better to provide more information than your doctor needs than to take a chance that you may skip an essential piece of your history.

People do not actually see themselves faint. And some individuals have a type of amnesia after they faint. They may be unable to recall very much about the episode—may even deny that they ever lost consciousness. If they do remember the faint, their recollection may not be accurate. When you go for your doctor's appointment, you may find it very helpful to bring along someone who has been with you when you fainted. This person can provide an eyewitness account of exactly what happened. For example, he or she may be able to describe how you looked before you fainted. Were you pale and/or sweating? Did you have convulsions?

In Chapter 5, there was a list of typical symptoms for people with orthostatic intolerance. The list came from a group of researchers who evaluated 90 individuals with symptomatic orthostatic intolerance to identify the symptoms that were present and to see which were the most common. Table 10-1, which shows how often these symptoms occurred in this group, may help you make your own symptom list.

Does all of this information really help? It certainly does! If you report that your fainting spells appear to be triggered by emotions or fatigue, for example, your doctor may immediately suspect neurocardiogenic syncope. When you lose consciousness suddenly, with no "prefaint" warning symptoms, this may suggest an irregular heart rhythm as the culprit. What if your faint comes on gradually and you do not recover very quickly? Your doctor may want to check for low blood sugar (hypoglycemia), hyperventilation (abnormally fast breathing), alcohol use, or medications (prescribed or otherwise). If you suddenly faint when you get up from a lying position, your doctor will most probably want to pursue a possible diagnosis of orthostatic hypotension.

Helpful as your history may be, the symptoms you report usually are not specific enough to provide the basis for a definite diagnosis. They are clues—important clues—in a larger puzzle.

Table 10-1 Common symptoms of orthostatic intolerance.

The Following Symptoms ...	Occurred in ... (%)
Lightheadedness (dizziness)	88
Weakness or tiredness	72
Trouble thinking or concentrating	47
Blurred vision	47
Tremulousness (involuntary trembling or quivering)	38
Vertigo (sensation that you or things around you are revolving or spinning)	37
Pallor (loss of color, or paleness)	31
Anxiety	29
Tachycardia (rapid heartbeat) or palpitations	26
Clammy feeling	19
Nausea	18

Adapted from Low PA, Suarez GA, Benarroch EC. Clinical autonomic disorders: Classification and clinical evaluation. In: Low PA, ed. *Clinical Autonomic Disorders*, 2nd edition. Philadelphia: Lippincott-Raven Publishers, 1997.

Your physical examination

The physical examination is a basic part of making an accurate diagnosis. Sometimes your physical appearance can point your doctor in the right direction. If you are abnormally pale, for example, this may suggest anemia (low red cell count in your blood, which reduces the amount of oxygen being transported) or blood loss, both of which can cause fainting. If you are pale only during the fainting episode itself, this may suggest that you have neurocardiogenic syncope.

Since fainting is the symptom that caused you to seek medical help, your doctor will pay special attention to possible abnormalities of your cardiovascular system and diseases and evaluation of your nervous system.

Measuring your blood pressure

Having your blood pressure measured is a routine part of just about every medical appointment. However, when you seek help for fainting, blood pressure readings take on a new importance. You can expect to have your blood pressure measured several times and while you are in various positions. Your doctor will take blood pressure readings when you are lying down (supine), sitting up, and then standing. Standing blood pressures should be taken when you first stand up and when you have been on your feet several minutes. Automatic blood pressure monitors are useful in that they typically allow your heart rate to be measured at the same time as your blood pressure. It is important that you immediately report any symptoms you may be experiencing in the different positions. You especially need to warn the doctor and/or nurse so that you do not have a fainting spell and risk being injured in a fall.

If you have a low blood volume, your blood pressure should drop when you stand, quickly followed by an increase in heart rate. As you have previously seen, a decrease in blood volume drops the blood pressure, leading the heart to try to compensate by increasing the speed at which it contracts. If you have orthostatic hypotension, on the other hand, standing causes the blood pressure to drop, but the heart rate typically does not change very much, if at all. The exact pattern of your blood pressure and heart rate on standing should provide important clues to underlying conditions that may not yet have been diagnosed. As you will see in a later section, in order to avoid the risk of falling, it may be easier, and safer, to have your blood pressure and heart rate measured during a tilt-table test.

Evaluating your breathing

Some people faint because they hyperventilate—breathe too quickly and become breathless. If your breathing is quick and shallow, however, your doctor may suspect the presence of pneumonia or congestive heart failure as a cause of fainting.

Examining the functioning of your various body systems

First, your doctor will examine how your heart is functioning. At times, simply listening to your heartbeat may provide a valuable clue. For example, a heart murmur (abnormal sound heard during the heart beat) may suggest that you have aortic stenosis (see Chapter 9) or mitral valve prolapse (see Chapter 7), among other conditions.

Your nervous system may also be an important factor in your tendency to faint. The doctor will check for signs of
• motor problems, including tremor, rigidity, and abnormally slow movements,
• changes in your vision,
• weakness affecting only one side of your body, and
• changes in your mental status (in order to exclude degenerative disorders of the brain).
Examination of your lungs may reveal congestive heart failure or some other condition that can potentially cause fainting. Checking your abdomen is helpful—perhaps you have tenderness that may indicate an ulcer, which could potentially be a source of blood loss. Your doctor will test your stool for hidden (occult) blood. Remember that losing enough blood, even when it occurs without you knowing it, can result in a faint.

Although all of this information can help in diagnosis, other tests may be necessary to identify the underlying cause of your faint. Your personal doctor can conduct some of these tests—for others, you may be referred to a specialist.

Did you know?

In 25–35% of people who faint, the history and physical examination are enough to make the diagnosis. More than three-fourths of the people for whom a cause for fainting can be identified do not require further diagnostic tests.

Psychiatric causes for fainting

Studies have shown that a definite diagnosis cannot be found to explain fainting in about one-third of the people who seek help for this problem. Other research suggests that in up to one-fourth of the people for whom a diagnosis is not found, fainting may be a sign of a psychiatric disorder. If this is the case, your doctor will need to refer you to an appropriate mental health professional.

Dizziness and fainting are listed as symptoms for several psychiatric illnesses. They include

• somatization disorder, which consists of multiple unexplained physical complaints for which the person seeks medical attention;
• generalized anxiety, which is excessive anxiety and worry most all the time;
• panic attack disorder, which consists of a sense of impending doom and fear, combined with certain physical symptoms that are not due to a substance or to a medical condition;
• major depression, which consists of depressed mood, lack of pleasurable feelings, significant weight loss or gain, insomnia or excessive sleep, fatigue, among other symptoms.

Diagnostic tests for fainting

Tests cost money—this is one of the realities that cannot be avoided. Therefore, it is important that your doctor order only those tests most likely to yield a definite diagnosis. Unfortunately, there is no master list of tests that can be applied to all people. The tests your doctor chooses should reflect the clues that have been provided by your history and physical examination.

The bad news is that the underlying cause for your fainting may not be found, no matter how many tests are done. The good news is that many people for whom the underlying cause is not identified do not have a recurrence of their faint and they do not appear to have a long-term problem. This section includes a number of tests often used to try to identify the underlying cause of fainting. Because of its growing importance as a diagnostic tool in identifying underlying causes of fainting, tilt-table testing is discussed in detail the next section.

Blood tests

Blood tests often are not that useful when you are trying to identify the cause of fainting. A hemoglobin count—a measurement of the oxygen-carrying component in red blood cells—may indicate anemia or blood loss. However, this has been shown to be useful in only about 5% of patients being evaluated for fainting. If you are taking certain medications, such as digoxin, it might be helpful to measure the levels of the drug in your blood.

Electrocardiograms

An electrocardiogram (ECG, or EKG) is a simple, inexpensive test in which the electrical activity of your heart is recorded. Electrodes that are attached to

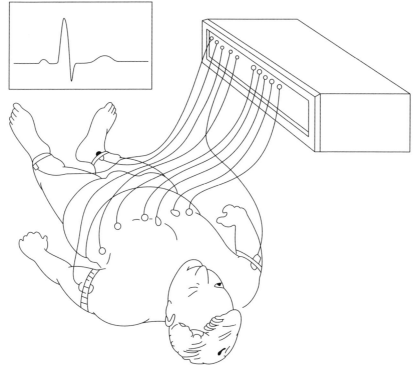

Figure 10-1 An ECG is a test in which the electrical activity of the heart is recorded. Electrodes that are attached to the body send impulses to a machine that prints out a graphic picture of the heart's activity.

your body send impulses to a machine that prints out a graphic picture of your heart's activity (see Figure 10-1). An ECG can usually be done in your doctor's office.

It is estimated that from 20% to 50% of patients will have an abnormal ECG. However, while an ECG may identify conditions such as atrial fibrillation, heart block (see Chapter 8), or a new or old heart attack, it typically does not provide a definite diagnosis of the underlying cause for fainting.

Holter monitoring

A Holter monitor is a portable ECG. Electrodes attached to your chest are connected to a small box that records your heart activity as you go about your daily activities. This provides your doctor with a round-the-clock record of your heart activity over several days.

One of the problems with abnormal heart rhythms is that they are likely to occur at odd times. You may have noticed that the strange sound your car engine is making always seems to mysteriously disappear the minute you try to describe it to a mechanic. The situation of trying to reproduce abnormal heart rhythms during an ECG is not that much different. This is one reason for the situation referred to in Chapter 1 in which your symptoms do not occur while you are being examined, leaving the doctor with the impression that you may be imagining them. A Holter monitor can be useful for diagnosing the disturbances in your heart's rhythm that occur at unpredictable times.

Your doctor will ask you to keep a record of your activities and any symptoms you experience while you are wearing the Holter monitor. Combining the information from the monitor and your activity-symptom log may allow your doctor to identify what activities caused changes in your heart rhythm and how this may have affected the appearance of symptoms. Of course, abnormalities in your heart rhythm do not always result in symptoms.

Holter monitoring is most likely to be used in individuals who have had frequent fainting episodes or related symptoms over a short period of time. It has the advantage of being automatic, that is, the wearer is not required to do anything.

Endless-loop recorders or event recorders

Endless-loop or event recorders are now considered better choices than a Holter monitor in many people being evaluated for faints. These smaller recorders can be attached for weeks or months, during which they continuously record an ECG.

Let us see how they work. You lose consciousness while you are wearing an endless-loop or event recorder. Upon awakening, you must press a button to automatically save the readings during the previous period, which reflect the time before and during your actual faint. Then, the ECG of your heart activity during the episode can be transmitted over the phone to a reference laboratory.

The endless-loop or event recorder allows your doctor the long-term opportunity to compare your symptoms with your heart rhythm at the time. Of course, in order to benefit from an endless-loop or event monitor, you must learn how to use it properly.

Implantable loop recorders

Going one step further, people who faint often may benefit from an implantable loop recorder, which can continuously record heart rate and rhythm for up to 14 months. This device, which is smaller than a pack of gum, is inserted just beneath the skin in the upper chest in a brief outpatient procedure. In order to capture the ECG at the time of a faint, the device either records automatically or a pager-sized activator can be held over the implantable recorder and a button is pushed. The recorded ECG can then be downloaded to a computer at a later date.

Electrophysiological testing

ECGs may not be conclusive, especially in people who report symptoms such as dizziness, palpitations, and fainting. Since irregular heart rhythms—arrhythmias—are unpredictable and may occur only occasionally, they are difficult to diagnose. Electrophysiological (EP) testing is now often used to evaluate various arrhythmias.

EP testing is more complicated than an ECG and is performed in a special EP laboratory. It consists of inserting electrode catheters into blood vessels and running them into the heart. (Electrode catheters are slender, hollow tubes that are able to conduct an electric current.) The catheters measure how impulses are conducted from one area of the heart to another. The electrodes are sometimes used to trigger the abnormal heart rhythm that is causing your symptoms. This allows the doctor to see the underlying heart rhythm and observe your symptoms in a controlled and safe environment. The electrodes can also be used as a pacemaker, using a small electrical current to normalize heart rate.

EP testing is often used to evaluate sustained rapid contractions of the ventricles—ventricular tachycardia. It is less useful in the evaluation of an abnormally slow heart rate—bradycardia—or heart block. Of course, any invasive procedure carries some risk of problems or complications. Fortunately, cases of bruising, infection, blocking of the blood vessel where the wires were inserted, or damaging the heart with the electrodes are rare.

Tilt-table testing

Tilt-table testing has been used to evaluate the mechanisms that cause fainting since before the 1950s. However, the tilt-table test has been widely used to provoke fainting and evaluate its underlying mechanisms only since the mid-1980s. It is widely considered the de facto "gold standard" for evaluating the reflex mechanisms that may be the underlying cause of fainting.

What is tilt-table testing?

The purpose of the tilt-table test is to see what happens when your body is tilted—head up—from a horizontal position. This mimics your body's responses when you stand up from a position of lying on your back.

What typically happens in a tilt-table test is as follows:

• You are instructed not to eat or drink anything for a certain period prior to the test—the point being to prevent nausea. If there is a possibility that you may have substantially reduced your fluid volume while fasting, the doctor may order fluid replacement by intravenous (IV) administration. You do not want the test results to be affected by your having an artificially low blood volume.

• The test area should be quiet, dimly lit, and at a comfortable temperature.

• You lie on your back on a special tilt-table, which has a footboard support. The mechanized table can be moved from a horizontal to a slanted position smoothly and quickly. It typically will be calibrated to upright tilt angles of from 60 to 90 degrees (straight up and down—at a right angle to the floor). You will be asked to lie quietly for 20–45 minutes before the test to allow plenty of time for your body to adjust to lying flat on your back.

• Monitoring equipment is attached. This includes a heart monitor, a blood pressure cuff or finger recording device, and a device to measure oxygen

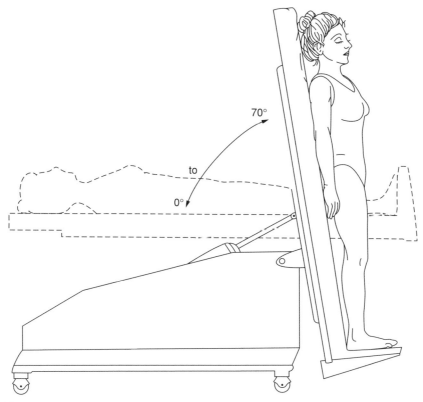

Figure 10-2 Tilt-table testing. The purpose of the tilt-table test is to see what happens when your body is tilted—head up—from a horizontal position. This mimics your body's responses when you stand up from a position of lying on your back.

saturation. Safety straps are applied across your chest and legs as a protection against your falling forward when you are being tilted up.

• The table is slowly raised to an angle of between 60 and 80 degrees—70 degrees now being the most common (see Figure 10-2). You are kept in this tilted position for 30–45 minutes.

• If you do not develop symptoms during this initial period of sustained tilt, your doctor may decide to add a provocation agent. What does this entail? First, you are usually returned to a flat, or supine, position for at least 10 minutes to reestablish your baseline readings. Provocation agents have effects that are similar to adrenalin (epinephrine). They increase your heart rate, much like exercise, and help show what occurs when your heart is beating faster. The drug may make your heart pound, which can be quite uncomfortable. However, the effects are temporary and will soon fade.

• The most commonly used provocation agent is isoproterenol, which is typically given by IV infusion. Other drugs sometimes used as provocation agents during tilt-table testing include nitroglycerin, edrophonium, adenosine triphosphate, epinephrine, and nitroprusside.

• There should be a nurse or laboratory technician who is experienced in tilt-table testing in attendance at all times during your test. A doctor should also be in attendance or immediately available if needed.

This amount of low-stress gravity should not be a problem for most people. However, individuals with different types of orthostatic intolerance will develop symptoms. For example, people with neurocardiogenic syncope will experience symptoms in association with a sudden fall in blood pressure and heart rate. Tilt-table testing is considered especially useful in identifying neurocardiogenic syncope as a cause of fainting in people 60 years of age and older.

While the various monitors are recording the objective data, it is up to you to provide subjective information. Tell the doctor and/or nurse when you are experiencing symptoms and if you feel like you are getting ready to pass out.

Once you have completed the test, someone else will need to drive you home. However, you should not have any restrictions on your activity, that is, you do not have to stay in bed or avoid any of your regular activities.

What can tilt-table testing show?

Someone who has an abnormal response to tilt-table testing typically shows one of five responses:

• *Classic neurocardiogenic response.* There is a sudden drop in blood pressure, typically followed quickly by a decrease in heart rate.

• *Dysautonomic response.* Dysautonomic indicates abnormal functioning of the autonomic nervous system (ANS). There is a gradual decrease in blood pressure to a level qualifying as hypotension, leading to a loss of consciousness. These individuals may show other signs of ANS malfunction, including sweating, constipation, and intolerance to heat.

• *Postural tachycardia syndrome (POTS) response.* The moderate fall in blood pressure is accompanied by an excessive increase in heart rate, which cannot compensate for an inability of the ANS to constrict the blood vessels to raise blood pressure.

• *Cerebral syncopal response.* Cerebral (brain) syncope is a fairly rare condition. It is associated with constriction of the blood vessels in the brain in the absence of slowed heartbeat and low blood pressure.

• *Psychogenic or psychosomatic (related to psychological causes) response.* In these individuals, there is no change in heart rate, blood pressure, brain wave recordings (electroencephalograms), or blood flow to the brain.

One of the easiest ways to understand the value of tilt-table testing is to actually see how responses between certain underlying causes of fainting differ. For example, Figure 10-3 shows what happens to blood pressure and heart rate when people with orthostatic hypotension (see Chapter 5), neurocardiogenic syncope (see Chapter 6), and POTS (see Chapter 7) undergo tilt-table testing.

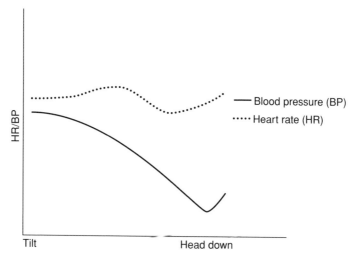

Figure 10-3 The typical tilt-table test response of someone with orthostatic hypotension.

Figure 10-3 shows the typical tilt-table test response of someone with orthostatic hypotension. In these people, there is a gradual fall in blood pressure, usually occurring within 10 minutes, but sometimes taking longer. Note that the heart rate stays about the same. As you may recall, orthostatic hypotension occurs because the ANS is not able to compensate for the drop in blood pressure when blood pools in the lower body upon standing. Therefore, the ANS neither constricts the blood vessels in the lower body nor increases heart rate—both of which would help increase blood pressure and avoid fainting. As you can see in this figure, the blood pressure begins to rise as soon as the table is returned to its original horizontal position, lowering the person's head.

Your doctor may also wish to have blood levels of the neurotransmitter norepinephrine measured during your tilt-table test in order to determine the presence and nature of ANS failure.

Figure 10-4 illustrates the usual response to tilt-table testing in people with neurocardiogenic syncope. Soon after the tilt-table is raised, the person experiences a drop in blood pressure. In someone with neurocardiogenic syncope, the first part of the response to this drop in blood pressure is normal—the ventricles begin to contract more strongly in an effort to pump more blood. The mechanism goes wrong since the mechanoreceptors in the walls of the ventricles misinterpret the strong contractions as a sign that the ventricle is too full. They send a message to the ANS to slow down the heart just the opposite of what would normally occur when blood pressure is low. This all happens in less time than it took you to read this description. Note in the illustration that the fall in heart rate actually occurs almost immediately after the initial drop in blood pressure. Again, as soon as the tilt-table is lowered to its horizontal position, both blood pressure and heart rate increase.

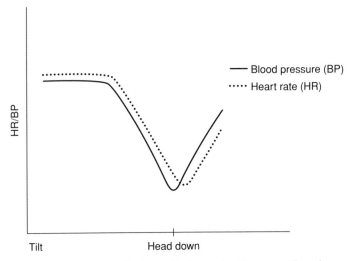

Figure 10-4 The usual response to tilt-table testing in people with neurocardiogenic syncope.

Figure 10-5, which shows you the response to tilt-table testing of a person with POTS, looks quite different from the other two. Remember that individuals suffering from POTS have an increase in heart rate of at least 30 beats per minute or a heart rate of at least 120 beats per minute occurring within the first 10 minutes of standing. The increase in heart rate may sometimes be associated with mild low blood pressure, as is shown in the illustration, but this is not

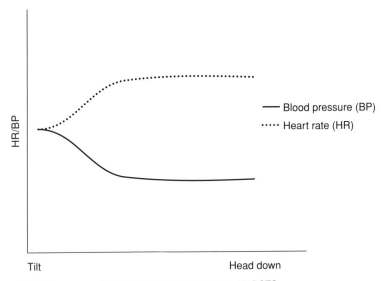

Figure 10-5 The response to tilt-table testing of a person with POTS.

always the case. The primary mechanism at work is an inability of the ANS to constrict the blood vessels in the lower body to increase blood return to the heart. This leads to the increase in heart rate as the heart tries to compensate for the decrease in blood reaching it. When the tilt-table is returned to its horizontal position, the blood pressure and heart rate do not immediately return to normal.

Who is a candidate for tilt-table testing?

Some guidelines have been developed to identify those people for whom tilt-table testing is indicated:
- People who have recurring episodes of fainting (1) without evidence of cardiovascular damage to the heart or blood vessels or (2) with evidence of this damage but when other causes of fainting have been ruled out.
- People who have had only one fainting episode but who are at high risk of injury. This group includes people who drive commercial vehicles, operate machinery, wash windows, work as commercial painters, perform surgery, fly planes, or compete in athletics, among others. Here again, there should either be no evidence of cardiovascular damage or, when structural cardiovascular disease is present, it should have been shown not to be responsible for the faint.
- People for whom an apparent cause of fainting has been established but who may also have neurocardiogenic syncope. When the presence of neurocardiogenic syncope in addition to the other diagnosis could affect treatment plans, further evaluation using tilt-table testing is justified.
- People with fainting episodes caused by or associated with exercise. Tilt-table testing may also be useful in other individuals
  - to differentiate between seizures and fainting accompanied by convulsions,
  - to evaluate people (especially older individuals) with recurring unexplained falls,
  - to assess recurring dizziness or presyncope (symptoms preceding a faint),
  - to evaluate unexplained faints in people with abnormal function of the peripheral nervous system, more especially the autonomic nervous system, and
  - as a follow-up evaluation to assess the success of therapy for neurocardiogenic syncope

A third category consists of conditions for which tilt-table testing is not now being used. However, some experts believe that this test may someday be used to evaluate people with
- recurring vertigo with no known cause
- recurring transient ischemic attacks
- chronic fatigue syndrome
- sudden infant death syndrome

The guidelines for using tilt-table testing currently specify two groups for which this test is not warranted. The first group includes people who have had only one fainting episode, who are not in a high-risk setting, and who clearly have symptoms of neurocardiogenic syncope. The second group consists of people with faints for which another cause has been established, and the presence of neurocardiogenic syncope would not change the treatment plan.

Looking forward...

Chapter 11 includes information about treating the fainting phenomenon. Some approaches deal directly with the most common mechanisms that contribute to fainting. Other treatment strategies are designed to correct the underlying cause for a faint.

References

Benditt DG, Ferguson DW, Grubb BP, et al. ACC expert consensus document. Tilt-table testing for assessing syncope. *Journal of the American College of Cardiology* 1996; 28:263–275.

Brignole M. Tilt table testing. In Grubb BP, Olshansky B, eds. *Syncope: Mechanisms and Management*. Malden, MA: Blackwell/Futura Publishing Co., Inc., 2005: 159–168.

Low PA, Suarez GA, Benarroch EE. Clinical autonomic disorders: classification and clinical evaluation. In: Low PA, ed. *Clinical Autonomic Disorders*, 2nd edition. Philadelphia: Lippincott-Raven Publishers, 1997.

Olshansky B. Syncope: Overview and approach to management. In: Grubb BP, Olshansky B, eds. *Syncope: Mechanisms and Management*. Malden, MA: Blackwell/Futura Publishing Co., Inc., 2005: 1–46.

CHAPTER 11

Treating fainting

As you have learned, fainting can have many different underlying causes, some of which can be very serious. It is vitally important that people who faint do *not* try to "self treat." Be sure to report any fainting episodes to your doctor so that you can be properly diagnosed and treated.

Because the underlying causes of fainting are so numerous, your doctor will have to select from among a number of approaches to treatment. And the chosen therapy would not exist in a vacuum. It will have to be compatible with treatments for any other medical conditions that are present.

Some underlying causes for fainting are obviously treatable. These include a low blood volume and blood loss. You might think that the answer to fainting due to a medication would be the simplest of all—just discontinue the medication. However, it is not always advisable or desirable to stop a medication even though it may contribute to orthostatic intolerance. Take Parkinson's disease, for example. People with Parkinson's disease typically cannot discontinue their medications if they are to have an acceptable quality of life. In this case, most doctors prefer to have their patients continue taking the medications for Parkinson's disease and then take measures to treat orthostatic hypotension separately.

A lot of factors will influence your doctor's approach to treatment. Take age, for instance. Adolescents who have episodes of fainting often outgrow the problem by the time they are in their twenties. Therefore, the doctor will choose a therapy to be used temporarily and then stopped. About 80% of adolescents who stop treatment after 1 or 2 years do not have recurrence of a problem. The remaining 20% will need to go back on therapy. Fainting is not usually a short-term problem in older people, however. Most of the older people with this problem have to continue therapy indefinitely.

Pregnancy can present some specific problems. At the time when a woman's blood volume increases by 50% during pregnancy, her ability to constrict the blood vessels in her lower body decreases. This can lead to a drop in blood pressure, which, if it is severe enough, can result in a faint. Of course, pregnant women should not use medications because they may affect the unborn child. Therefore, the doctor may be limited to recommending changes in everyday activities, such as using special support stockings and resting in bed.

In addition, the problem may not disappear upon delivery of the baby. A new mother may be at risk for fainting because her blood vessels are still expanded while her blood volume is returning to normal. This "postpartum syncope" is important because a fainting episode in a mother who is carrying her child can lead to serious injuries for both of them.

Making changes in everyday activities

One of your doctor's most important roles is to help educate you about what causes fainting and what you can do to help prevent it. For example, if you have symptoms before a fainting episode, learn to immediately squat or lie down to try to avoid the faint. Do not have someone hold you up so that you remain in a standing position. Just common sense? Of course. However, it is surprising how often the basic education of a patient who faints can be overlooked.

You might consider getting an automatic blood pressure and pulse monitor. Measure your blood pressure when you are lying down and when you are standing. Take your readings and record them at the same time each day. And be sure to check your blood pressure when you are having symptoms. It will also help your doctor if you record the number of minutes you are able to stand still before you begin to develop symptoms, especially if it is less than 10 minutes.

Story on salt (and water)

For years you have been bombarded on all sides by messages about the evils of eating too much salt. It is true that people with high blood pressure are advised to eat a diet that is restricted in the mineral sodium. The most common source of sodium in your diet is everyday table salt, or sodium chloride. So what is the problem?

Americans often apply the adage "if a little bit is good, a lot must be better" to too many situations. In the case of salt and sodium, the opposite may be true. While in general it may be a good idea not to eat a lot of salt, you can also have problems associated with unnecessarily cutting your intake of salt too much. Therefore, one of the first recommendations your doctor may make is for you to actually increase your intake of salt and water. These measures should help expand your blood volume, raise your blood pressure, and reduce your symptoms, including fainting. Also, keep in mind that hot weather and having a cold or the flu may require extra salt and water to avoid making your symptoms worse.

You may be able to increase your salt intake sufficiently by consuming salty foods. If you cannot get enough salt this way, your doctor may recommend that you take a salt tablet. Set up a water-drinking schedule to make sure you get enough fluid. Do not rely on feelings of thirst—they are not always reliable indicators of when and how much you need to be drinking. Watch for signs that you may be getting too much fluid, including trouble breathing or excessive swelling at your ankles. If either of these situations occurs, you will have to cut back on salt.

Watch your activities

Make it a practice to stand up slowly from a lying or seated position, especially when getting up in the morning. First, sit on the side of the bed for a few minutes before you try to stand up. If you are dizzy, sit back down for a few minutes.

Avoid prolonged periods of standing, especially standing quite still. Schedule most of your activities in the afternoon when blood pressure is higher rather than in the morning when it is at its lowest.

Try to stay up during the day—do not lie in bed. And sleep with your head elevated 5–20 degrees. One easy way to do this is to place bricks or blocks under the head of your bed to raise it 6–12 inches. This should reduce the amount of urinating you do overnight, decrease the sudden pooling of your blood upon arising, and reduce supine hypertension, that is, blood pressure that is too high when you are lying down. In addition, never lying completely flat may help your brain adjust to lower blood pressure. However, you may have to add a footboard to keep you from sliding off the bed. Keep in mind that tilting the head of your bed up may contribute to low blood pressure and leg cramps.

Keep yourself cool

Do not get overheated—keep cool during hot weather or in any other warm environment. Avoid hot showers or baths, which may dilate your blood vessels, making the return of blood to your heart more difficult. If possible, you may want to have a chair in your shower so that you can sit, when necessary.

Secrets of wise eating and drinking

Caffeine can increase blood pressure. People who have postprandial hypotension might try drinking a couple of cups of strong coffee about 30 minutes before a meal. However, the ability of caffeine to raise your blood pressure may decrease the longer you drink coffee or other caffeine-containing beverages. So, if your blood pressure tends to be lowest in the mornings, you might save your coffee drinking until before breakfast.

Try to avoid alcohol and large meals, which may cause vasodilation—enlargement of your blood vessels. Small, frequent meals are preferred. Do not stand up suddenly after a meal, especially one that has been high in carbohydrates (sugars and starches).

No strain, your gain

Mild exercise should help your veins return blood from your lower body to your heart. Remember that the contraction and relaxation of your leg muscles "milks" veins, pushing the blood upward against gravity. However, you may need to avoid vigorous exercise if this tends to bring on orthostatic hypotension. Schedule your exercise at a time of day when your blood pressure is higher. Swimming may be a good choice for someone with failure of the autonomic nervous system (ANS) since the pressure of the water may act like a compression garment and help counteract low blood pressure.

Avoid activities that involve straining, which may decrease the blood flow from your lower body through your chest to your heart. This means that you should avoid lifting heavy objects. Of course, you cannot avoid urinating or passing stool just try not to strain during these activities. Men may benefit from sitting while they urinate.

Clothes that hug
Sometimes the doctor may recommend some type of clothing to decrease pooling of blood in the veins in your lower body and to increase the pressure on your lower body, thereby helping return blood to your heart. Probably the best known of these are Jobst stockings, which are like an elasticized leotard that should reach to the waist. Most of the pressure is exerted at the ankles, with much less pressure at the waist. The disadvantages of compressive stockings are that they are expensive, hot, and can be difficult to put on.

Did you know?

Air-filled antigravity suits that are used by the astronauts are a type of counterpressure suit that would probably be useful for people who have problems with blood pooling when they stand. However, this would be a cost that no insurance carrier would allow!

Making the right moves
Doctors have developed exercises that may help you increase your blood pressure. Table 11-1 describes some special physical activities that can help you reduce orthostatic hypotension and its symptoms.

Monitoring your medications

Whenever possible, your doctor will change your prescription from a drug that can cause fainting to one that does not. Drugs for high blood pressure and other heart medications are likely culprits. Do not stop any of your medications on your own; this must be approved by your doctor!

Remember that a number of different medications and substances can cause fainting. They include
- alcohol,
- beta-blockers, which are used primarily to treat high blood pressure,
- vasodilating drugs such as hydralazine, which are used to treat high blood pressure among other conditions,
- drugs that decrease or block the peripheral activities of the sympathetic nervous system (peripherally acting antiadrenergics) such as prazosin or reserpine, which are used to treat high blood pressure,
- tricyclic antidepressants,
- L-dopa, which is used to treat Parkinson's disease,

Table 11-1 Exercises to help reduce the symptoms of orthostatic hypotension.

Physical Maneuver	What to Do*
Squatting	Move from a standing position to a squatting position
Genuflecting/contracting	Move from a standing position to kneeling on one knee. Then shift your body forward and backward at the waist while continuing to kneel
Leg crossing	While standing, cross the right foot over the left and contract your leg muscles; repeat with the other foot
Knee flexing	While standing, march in place
Toe raising	While standing, raise up on the front portion of your feet and contract your calf muscles for 5–10 seconds. Return your feet flat to floor and rhythmically repeat the cycle
Neck flexing	While standing, touch your chin to your chest and tighten the muscles in your neck.
Abdominal contracting	While standing, isometrically[†] contract the abdominal muscles
Thigh contracting	While standing, isometrically[†] contract the muscles at the front of your thigh
Combination	Perform those maneuvers that seem to decrease your symptoms of orthostatic hypotension in combinations-for example, neck flexing and abdominal contracting

* During all exercises, avoid Valsalva straining, that is, forcibly exhaling when your mouth is closed and nose is blocked (like the maneuver you do to pop open your ears when you are flying), since it increases the pressure in your chest and cuts down the blood flow to your heart.
[†] Isometrically implies contracting a muscle without shortening its length.
Source: Adapted from Bouvette, et al. *Mayo Clinic Proceedings* 1996;71:847–853.

- calcium-channel blockers, which are used to treat high blood pressure and angina (heart-related chest pain),
- angiotensin-converting enzyme inhibitors, which are used to treat high blood pressure and congestive heart failure,
- methyldopa, which is used to treat high blood pressure,
- barbiturates, which are used as sedatives, for insomnia, and to control epileptic seizures, among other uses,
- anesthetics, which act on the central nervous system (CNS) to cause sleep before invasive procedures, including surgery,
- diuretics, which are used to treat high blood pressure and reduce fluid retention in congestive heart failure,
- opiates, which contain opium or one of its derivatives and are used as sedative narcotics,
- bromocriptine, which is used to treat Parkinson's disease and female infertility, among other conditions,
- phenothiazines, which are used as tranquilizers in the treatment of psychiatric disorders, and
- nitrates, which are used to relieve the pain of angina or heart attack.

In addition, there are a number of over-the-counter (OTC) products that may raise your blood pressure. When your blood pressure is high, you may be more likely to experience enough of a drop upon standing to cause symptoms of orthostatic intolerance. Be sure to check with your doctor before you take OTC cold medications, diet pills, nose drops and sprays, and/or eye drops.

Nondrug treatments

This section reviews three nondrug treatments that are useful in some people who faint. Two of the procedures, head-up tilt training and biofeedback, are noninvasive. Pacing and implantable defibrillators are invasive, meaning that they require surgery.

Head-up tilt training

Note that the tilt-table testing (see Chapter 10) used to identify different underlying causes of fainting can sometimes also be a treatment. This therapy came about after researchers wondered if exposing the cardiovascular system of someone with neurocardiogenic syncope to repeated and prolonged periods of head-up tilt might be of benefit.

Individuals who use head-up tilt training are first head-up tilted for increasingly long periods of time on the same type of tilt-table used for evaluation. Once they are able to get through a session of a determined length without symptoms, it is time to try it at home. Since people typically do not have their own tilt-tables, they train by standing against a wall for 30 minutes or more, once or twice a day. In some people, this results in a complete disappearance of the fainting episodes (Ector et al., 1998).

Biofeedback

As you recall, some people faint in certain recognized situations, such as when they see blood or even catch sight of a needle. In these individuals, biofeedback has been successful in helping them to become desensitized to the psychological trigger for their episodes.

Pacing and defibrillation

Pacing is the insertion of an artificial pacemaker to stimulate or regulate the heart's contractions. The pacemaker replaces your heart's sinoatrial node, sending tiny electrical impulses to the heart muscle. A pacemaker is prescribed typically for someone who has a slow or an irregular heartbeat. Pacing is highly effective in people who faint as the result of sick sinus syndrome or atrioventricular block (see Chapter 8).

Permanent pacing is perhaps one of the most controversial treatments for neurocardiogenic syncope. Although, pacing is most likely to be considered for those people with neurocardiogenic syncope or orthostatic hypotension who have a significant slowing of heart rate and even asystole (heart stops contracting), researchers have come to vastly different conclusions about its value in these individuals. One important point to remember is that in people with neurocardiogenic syncope, the drop in blood pressure occurs before heart rate slows. Therefore, the ability of a pacemaker to prevent the slowing of the heart rate would not actually prevent the low blood pressure and the resulting faint (Sra and Akhtar, 1995). Pacemakers are being developed that are able to sense drops in blood pressure and then start pacing at an earlier point in the process compared to existing units.

Some doctors felt that it was a good idea to perform a tilt-table test in which the person has a temporary pacemaker in place to see if it is effective in solving the underlying problem; however this is seldom done today. Implantable loop recorders are now used to detect slow heart rates during episodes of syncope. At best, pacing should not be used until other measures have failed. In most cases, some type of drug therapy must be used in addition to the pacemaker.

If you have a fast heartbeat (ventricular tachycardia or fibrillation), the doctor may recommend insertion of an implantable defibrillator. The implantable defibrillator automatically senses when your heart goes out of rhythm and shocks it to restore normal heart rhythm. Frequently, pacemakers are now built into implantable defibrillators.

Common drug treatments

There are a number of factors that may influence your doctor's choice of a medication to treat your fainting. In some cases, two or more medications may be necessary to satisfactorily control your tendency to faint.

The most common pharmacological approach to treating orthostatic hypotension is midodrine and/or fludrocortisone. Individuals with neurocardiogenic syncope and postural tachycardia syndrome (POTS) are typically treated with midodrine, fludrocortisone (and salt), and/or beta-blocking drugs (Bloomfield et al., 1999).

Midodrine

Midodrine is the only drug approved by the US Food and Drug Administration for the treatment of orthostatic hypotension.

It is also used to treat neurocardiogenic syncope and POTS. This alpha-1 agonist increases blood pressure by constricting your blood vessels, particularly arterioles (small arteries) and veins. It has the advantage of not stimulating your heart, and, since it does not cross the blood–brain barrier, it does not stimulate your CNS. Side effects of midodrine therapy may include
- a feeling of your hair standing on end ("piloerection"),
- dilation of your pupils,
- goose bumps,
- tingling,
- itching, especially of the scalp,
- supine hypertension, and
- possible nausea.

One particular advantage of midodrine is that it begins to have an effect soon after you take it. In addition, it is short acting, thus dosing can be tailored to fit your activities each day. For example, if you know you are not going to be standing for the next few hours, you might be able to skip a dose. By avoiding use of midodrine after 6 p.m., the risk of supine hypertension at night is minimized.

Several studies (Jankovic et al., 1993; Low et al., 1997) have shown that midodrine improved orthostatic hypotension associated with failure of the ANS. Compared to a placebo, midodrine improved dizziness/lightheadedness, weakness/fatigue, fainting, low energy level, impaired ability to stand, and feeling of depression. The midodrine group had only a slightly higher incidence of side effects, which included itching and tingling scalp, high blood pressure when lying down, and urgent feelings of needing to urinate.

Research has also shown that midodrine is effective in people suffering from neurocardiogenic syncope and POTS. In one study (Ward et al., 1998), researchers found that midodrine reduced symptoms of neurocardiogenic syncope and improved the participants' quality of life.

If you are taking midodrine, make sure you follow your doctor's directions about increasing your intake of salt and water. At times, midodrine may not appear to be effective when the real problem is an insufficient amount of blood available to support normal blood pressure.

Fludrocortisone

Fludrocortisone is a mineralocorticoid that increases blood pressure by expanding blood volume and making your blood vessels more sensitive to the constrictive effects of norepinephrine. In order for fludrocortisone to work effectively, you need to increase your intake of salt and water.

Fludrocortisone is commonly used in younger people with neurocardiogenic syncope or orthostatic hypotension. It is often combined with other agents, such as midodrine and/or beta-blockers. Fludrocortisone is not as well tolerated in older individuals, especially for long-term treatment (Hussain et al., 1996).

Fludrocortisone therapy may increase your risk of
• low potassium and magnesium levels in your blood due to excessive loss in urine,
• swelling in your legs and feet from fluid retention,
• weight gain,
• headache,
• supine hypertension,
• enlargement of the heart, and
• congestive heart failure.
In addition, if you already have migraines or acne, fludrocortisone may make these conditions worse. A few people report some hair loss associated with this drug.

If your doctor prescribes a potassium supplement to help prevent low blood levels of this important mineral, be sure you take it! When potassium levels drop too low, you may experience muscle weakness, fatigue, and muscle pain or tenderness.

Keep in mind that fludrocortisone does not act immediately. And, once it has expanded your fluid volume, the effect will last for awhile after you have stopped taking the medication. This means that if you do develop negative side effects from the fluid expansion, there will be a time lag between the time you stop taking the medication and the disappearance of the effects.

Beta-blocking drugs

Beta-blockers typically are used to treat high blood pressure, irregularities in the timing of ventricular contractions, and angina (heartrelated chest pain). However, these agents are also thought to reduce the strength of contractions of your heart. In people with neurocardiogenic syncope, this allows the mechanoreceptors to stop sending the brain the inaccurate message that the blood pressure is too high, which causes the sympathetic nervous system to further decrease blood pressure by slowing the heart and expanding blood vessels.

Beta-blockers, such as propranolol, metoprolol, pindolol, and atenolol, may be useful in some individuals with neurocardiogenic syncope or POTS. However, it is important to note that they are not useful—in fact, may even be harmful—in people with orthostatic hypotension. Negative side effects of beta-blockers can include low blood pressure, slowed heart rate, fatigue, congestive heart failure, and impotence. Beta-blockers can sometimes actually increase your risk of fainting. Recent studies have suggested that they are more helpful in older patients (more than 42 yrs of age) than in younger patients.

Other drugs used to treat fainting

Researchers have investigated a number of other drugs to see if they might be useful in preventing fainting. They may sometimes be used in combination with midodrine, fludrocortisone, and/or beta-blockers.

Selective serotonin reuptake inhibitors

As you saw in Chapter 6, a higher level of serotonin inhibits the passage of sympathetic impulses from one nerve cell to another. So an agent that inhibits the reuptake of serotonin by its receptors—a selective serotonin reuptake inhibitor (SSRI)—causes larger amounts of the neurotransmitter to remain available in the synapse. SSRIs are typically used as antidepressants.

It is thought that SSRIs, such as sertraline, fluoxetine, and paroxetine, may help prevent neurocardiogenic syncope because they reduce the sympathetic impulses that signal the heart to contract more strongly. This, in turn, reduces the misinformation the mechanoreceptors are sending to the brain, which is triggering the inappropriate decrease in heart rate and vasoconstriction. Some studies have shown that up to half of the people with neurocardiogenic syncope who had not responded to other treatments benefited from this agent. Sertraline has also been found to be beneficial in preventing recurring neurocardiogenic

syncope in children and in adolescents who did not respond to other medications (Grubb et al., 1994; Lenk et al., 1997). Another SSRI, fluoxetine, has been
used successfully to treat neurocardiogenic syncope in individuals who had
not been able to prevent symptoms on other forms of therapy (Grubb et al.,
1993). In a recent randomized, double-blind, placebo-controlled study, paroxetine was found to significantly improve symptoms of people with neurocardiogenic syncope who had not responded to or could not take other medications
(Di Girolamo et al., 1999). Researchers have also had some success in treating
patients with orthostatic hypotension with the SSRIs venlafaxine, fluoxetine,
and nefazodone.

Possible side effects of therapy with SSRIs may include nausea, dry mouth,
agitation, diarrhea, loss of appetite, insomnia, or drowsiness and sleepiness.
Some SSRIs are known to cause high blood pressure.

Pyridostigmine

Pyridostigine inhibits the breakdown of a compound known as acetylcholine,
a critical component of normal autonomic nerve function. The ganglia (i.e.,
junctions) of both the sympathetic and parasympathetic nervous systems use
acetylcholine to function. The drug was originally used to treat a muscle paralysis disorder called myasthenia gravis. However, recent studies have shown
that the drug is remarkably effective in preventing drops in blood pressure
while standing, without causing excessive elevations in blood pressure while
lying down. The drug has been effective in both orthostatic hypotension and
POTS (Raj, 2005; Singer et al., 2003, 2006). The principal side effects of pryi-
dostigmine are upset stomach, diarrhea, and cramping.

Disopyramide

Disopyramide works to correct irregular heartbeat and is used for high blood
pressure, tachycardia, and angina (heart-related chest pain), among other conditions. There are differing reports of the usefulness of this drug in treating
neurocardiogenic syncope. Possible side effects of disopyramide include dry
mouth, blurred vision, and urinary retention.

Theophylline

Theophylline is a bronchodilator—a drug that opens bronchial air passages
(main branches of the windpipe, leading into the lungs). These drugs are used
primarily to treat bronchial asthma and other lung conditions. Since one of its
effects is to increase vasoconstriction, theophylline is sometimes used to treat
neurocardiogenic syncope. Once in a while, theophylline may be used to treat
someone who faints as the result of sick sinus syndrome.

Unfortunately, in order to have the desired effect, doses of theophylline must
be large and are not usually well tolerated. Possible side effects of this drug
include nausea, tremor, and stimulation of the CNS.

Methylphenidate

Methylphenidate stimulates the CNS and causes vasoconstriction. It increases the release of the neurotransmitters norepinephrine and dopamine in the part of the nervous system that affects body posture and reflex mechanisms.

Use of this drug is usually limited because of its potential side effects, which can include agitation, tremor, insomnia, headache, nausea, and high blood pressure when you are lying down (supine hypertension). Methylphenidate can also be habit forming, that is, you are at risk of becoming dependent on the drug.

Erythropoietin

Erythropoietin is a hormone that is involved in the control of red cell production for your blood. It may be used in cases where fainting is caused by anemia and other measures have failed to correct the situation. This drug has also been effective in improving orthostatic tolerance in people with autonomic failure, who may often be anemic.

Erythropoietin must be given by injection, and there may be burning at the site. Potential side effects include high blood pressure, which can contribute to problems in the brain, headache, coldness, sweating, bone pain, and seizures.

Pseudoephedrine and ephedrine

Pseudoephedrine is used primarily as a nasal decongestant in both prescription and OTC products. Some researchers have reported that it is effective in the treatment of neurocardiogenic syncope, especially in children. When people are treated with this drug, however, their response very quickly begins to decrease—that is, they build up a tolerance to it. It also has the side effect of stimulating the CNS.

Ephedrine is sometimes used to treat orthostatic hypotension. Possible side effects include rapid heart rate, tremor, and supine hypertension.

Clonidine

Clonidine is an alpha-2 adrenergic agonist. What this means is that it acts to inhibit sympathetic outflow, which can result in low blood pressure. However, clonidine can sometimes be used to treat orthostatic hypotension in people with severe autonomic failure who have little or no remaining sympathetic activity. Common problems with this drug include dry mouth, slowed heart rate, and low blood pressure due to the slowed heart rate.

Yohimbine

Yohimbine works as a "sympathetic stimulator," meaning that it helps your own sympathetic impulses increase vasoconstriction. It increases blood pressure by causing a small increase in blood norepinephrine levels. Although research has not provided consistent evidence of yohimbine's value in treating fainting, it is sometimes used in people with orthostatic hypotension.

In at least one study, yohimbine decreased orthostatic intolerance in a small number of people with neurocardiogenic syncope (Mosqueda-Garcia et al., 1998). However, in a study (Senard et al., 1993) of people with Parkinson's disease who had orthostatic hypotension, researchers found that yohimbine was not effective in increasing blood pressure.

Side effects of yohimbine can include anxiety, nervousness, and diarrhea.

Looking forward . . .

Chapter 12 will include a few final thoughts on fainting and provide some insight into the philosophy of a doctor specializing in the treatment of patients who suffer from the fainting phenomenon.

References

Benditt DG, Sutton R. Bradyarrhythmias as a cause of syncope. In: Grubb BP, Olshansky B, eds. *Syncope: Mechanisms and Management*. Malden, MA: Blackwell/Futura Publishing Co., Inc., 2005: 92–120.

Bloomfield DM, Sheldon R, Grubb BP, et al. Panel consensus. Putting it together: A new treatment algorithm for vasovagal syncope and related disorders. *American Journal of Cardiology* 1999;84:33Q–39Q.

Bouvette CM, McPhee BR, Opfer-Gehrking TL, et al. Role of physical counter-maneuvers in the management of orthostatic hypotension: Efficacy and biofeedback augmentation. *Mayo Clinic Proceedings* 1996;71:847–853.

Di Girolamo E, Di Iorio C, Sabatini P, et al. Effects of paroxetine hydrochloride, a selective serotonin reuptake inhibitor, on refractory vasovagal syncope: A randomized, double-blind, placebo-controlled study. *Journal of the American College of Cardiology* 1999;33:1227–1230.

Ector H, Reybrouck T, Heidbüchel H, et al. Tilt training: A new treatment for recurrent neurocardiogenic syncope and severe orthostatic intolerance. *PACE* 1998;21:193–196.

Gazit Y, Nahir M, Grahame R, et al. Dysautonomia in the joint hypermobility syndrome. *American Journal of Medicine* 2003;115:33–40.

Grubb BP. Dysautonomic (orthostatic) syncope. In: Grubb BP, Olshansky B, eds. *Syncope: Mechanisms and Management*. Armonk, NY: Futura Publishing Co., Inc., 2005: 72–91.

Grubb BP. Neurocardiogenic syncope. In: Grubb BP, Olshansky B, eds. *Syncope: Mechanisms and Management*. Armonk, NY: Futura Publishing Co., Inc., 1998: 73–106.

Grubb BP, Kanjwal Y, Kosinski D. The postural tachycardia syndrome: a concise guide to diagnosis and management *Journal of Cardiac Electrophysiology* 2006;17:108–112.

Grubb BP, Karas B. Diagnosis and management of neurocardiogenic syncope. *Current Opinions in Cardiology* 1998;13:29–35.

Grubb BP, Samoil D, Kosinski D, et al. Use of sertraline hydrochloride in the treatment of refractory neurocardiogenic syncope in children and adolescents. *Journal of the American College of Cardiology* 1994;24:490–494.

Grubb BP, Wolfe DA, Samoil D, et al. Usefulness of fluoxetine hydrochloride for prevention of resistant upright tilt-induced syncope. *PACE* 1993;16:458–464.

Hussain RM, McIntosh SJ, Lawson J, et al. Fludrocortisone in the treatment of hypotensive disorders in the elderly. *Heart* 1996;76:507–509.

Jankovic J, Gilden JL, Hiner BC, et al. Neurogenic orthostatic hypotension: A double-blind, placebo-controlled study with midodrine. *The American Journal of Medicine* 1993;95: 38–48.

Lenk M, Alehan D, Ozme S, et al. The role of serotonin re-uptake inhibitors in preventing recurrent unexplained childhood syncope: A preliminary review. *European Journal of Pediatrics* 1997;156:747–750.

Lipsitz LA, Marks ER, Koestner J, et al. Reduced susceptibility to syncope during postural tilt in old age. Is beta-blockade protective? *Archives of Internal Medicine* 1989;149:2709–2712.

Low PA, Gilden JL, Freeman R, et al. Efficacy of midodrine vs. placebo in neurogenic orthostatic hypotension. *JAMA* 1997;13:1046–1051.

Mosqueda-Garcia R, Furlan R, Tank J, et al. The elusive pathophysiology of neurally-mediated syncope. *Circulation* 2000;102:2898–2906.

Raj SR, Black BK, Biaggioni I, et al. Acetylcholinertorse inhibition improves tachycardia in Postural tachycardia syndrome. *Circulation* 2005;111:2734–3740.

Senard JM, Rascol O, Rascol A, et al. Lack of yohimbine effect on ambulatory blood pressure recording: A double-blind crossover trial in Parkinsonians with orthostatic hypotension. *Fundamentals of Clinical Pharmacology* 1993;7:465–470.

Singer W, Opfer-gehrking TL, McPhee BR, et al. Acetylcholinerase inhibition: A normal approach in the treatment of neurogenic orthostatic hypotension. *Journal of Neurology Neurosurgery and Psychiatry* 2003;74:1294–1298.

Singer W, Sanchoni P, Opfer-Gehrking TL, et al. Pyridostymine treatment trial in neurogenic orthostatic hypotension. *Arch Neurol* 2006;63:515–518.

Sra JS, Akhtar M. Cardiac pacing during neurocardiogenic (vasovagal) syncope. *Journal of Cardiovascular Electrophysiology* 1995;6:751–760.

Stumpf JL, Mitrzyk B. Management of orthostatic hypotension. *American Journal of Hospital Pharmacy* 1994;51:648–660.

Ward CR, Gray JC, Gilroy JJ, et al. Midodrine: A role in the management of neurocardiogenic syncope. *Heart* 1998;79:45–49.

CHAPTER 12

Wrapping up . . .

Recurring episodes of unexplained fainting are both common and frustrating. Fainting may be a symptom of a serious disorder or simply indicate a relatively harmless condition. The wide variety of conditions that can result in fainting makes it essential that you seek out trained medical advice.

Take fainting seriously. Even if the underlying cause for your fainting turns out to be basically harmless, any sudden loss of consciousness can lead to a fall, which may result in serious injury. Fainting or near-fainting spells while driving can have disastrous consequences. And there is more than the risk of physical injury at stake. At times, the most difficult aspect of this type of condition is the social disruption it can cause. Many people who suffer from recurrent fainting have severe problems with school, employment, and/or family relations.

You and your doctor are in a two-way partnership. It falls upon you to be a detailed and complete reporter, providing as much information as possible concerning your fainting episodes. For example, exactly what occurs before, during, and after a fainting episode can provide valuable clues to your diagnosis. Volunteer information that you think may be relevant. Do not make your doctor probe for every little detail.

In turn, your doctor must be a thorough and careful detective, following the clues provided by your medical history, your report of what occurs when you faint, and the diagnostic testing that is performed. While diagnosing most causes of fainting is fairly straightforward, some cases are more complicated and require in-depth investigation. Keep in mind that there are hundreds of possible underlying causes of fainting—a considerable diagnostic challenge for the best of physicians.

There are times when, in spite of everyone's best efforts, the exact cause of fainting may not be discovered. This is not the fault of you or your doctor. Medical technology and science have not yet progressed to a point where each and every disorder can be identified. Also, there are probably many conditions not yet recognized as a cause of fainting. Even when a diagnosis has been established, treatment may be difficult and require several attempts at medical therapy. There are times when a doctor will exhaust all of the usual treatment options. In these instances, you may need to be referred to a medical center that specializes in caring for people whose disorders are more difficult to treat.

Therapy is sometimes very straightforward; at other times, it can be quite involved. And, as you grow older, your therapy may need to be altered to meet your ever-changing needs. Whether simple or complicated, successful treatment requires a team effort between you and your doctor. You, in turn, will need support from your family and friends. The factors that best predict successful treatment are a determined patient and a supportive family and/or social environment.

Many times illnesses—particularly those of the autonomic nervous system (ANS)—may not be life-threatening, but they still represent life-altering problems. Many people find it difficult to adjust to the fact that their lives are not quite what they had anticipated. Individuals who suffer from chronic conditions that cause fainting sometimes find it helpful to obtain counseling for themselves and their family members.

Many autonomic disorders are chronic, meaning that they cannot be cured. It is difficult to live with a chronic condition of any type, and these disorders are no exception. However, bothersome symptoms can often be controlled, in much the same way as they are in asthma or epilepsy. If your symptoms are adequately controlled, you can live a relatively normal life with only minor restrictions.

As time goes on, the ability of doctors to diagnose and treat these disorders will improve. Current technological advances in genetics, molecular biology, and diagnostic imaging are now being applied to the different disorders that cause recurrent fainting, such as postural tachycardia syndrome. These advances will give doctors increasingly better ways to recognize, diagnose, and treat these various disorders.

Since information in the fields of fainting and disorders of the ANS is always growing, it is sometimes difficult to keep up to date. The following websites are good sources of accurate information:

National Dysautonomia Research Foundation www.ndrf.org
Heart Rhythm Society www.hrspatient.org
Sudden Arrhythmia Death Syndromes www.sads.org/main.html
Dysautonomia Youth Network of America www.dynakids.org
Dysautonomia Information Network www.dinet.org
Syncope Trust and Anoxic Reflex Seizure Group www.stars.org.uk

Glossary of useful terms

Abdominal aorta: The abdominal aorta is that part of your descending aorta that is the origin of arteries in your abdomen.

Acetylcholine: Acetylcholine is a neurotransmitter found in your brain, autonomic nervous system (ANS), and in all neuromuscular junctions (tiny gaps between neurons and the muscles they stimulate). It slows the heart rate and stimulates the contraction of skeletal muscles.

Action potential: Action potential refers to the process by which the electrical charge of the outer membrane of a nerve cell, or neuron, undergoes changes that allow impulses to travel along the neuron and, therefore, along your nerves.

Addison's disease: Addison's disease is a partial or total failure of the cortex of the adrenal glands. It is characterized by a bronze coloration of the skin, anemia, weakness, nausea, and low blood pressure.

Adrenal glands: You have two adrenal glands, one located above each kidney. In regard to blood pressure control, the adrenal glands produce the hormone neurotransmitters epinephrine and norepinephrine (which affect heart rate and blood pressure) and mineralocorticoids (which affect fluid balance).

Afferent neuron: See sensory neuron.

Aldosterone: Aldosterone is a hormone secreted by the adrenal glands. It causes your kidneys to retain sodium and water, which raises blood pressure.

Alpha-blocking agents: Alpha-blocking agents cause dilation of peripheral blood vessels, which lowers peripheral resistance and reduces blood pressure.

Amnesia: Amnesia is a loss or impairment of memory.

Amyloidosis: Amyloidosis is a group of disorders in which insoluble proteins, called amyloid, accumulate in body tissues and impair their function.

Anemia: Anemia is a deficiency in the oxygen-carrying component of the blood.

Angiotensin: Angiotensin is a general term for a group of hormones that act as vasoconstrictors.

Angiotensin-converting enzyme inhibitor (ACE): ACE inhibitors lower blood pressure by preventing both constriction of your arterioles and retention of sodium and fluid in your kidneys.

Anorexia: In this instance, anorexia refers to anorexia nervosa, an eating disorder characterized by fear of obesity, abnormal body image, and prolonged refusal to eat, which leads to starvation and even death.

Aorta: The aorta is the large, main artery in the body. With the exception of the pulmonary arteries, all of the arteries of the body branch off from the aorta.

Aortic stenosis: Aortic stenosis is an abnormal narrowing of the aortic valve, which is the semilunar valve between the left ventricle of the heart and the ascending aorta. Aortic stenosis limits the amount of blood that the left ventricle can eject with each contraction, thereby reducing the blood available for systemic circulation.

Arch of the aorta: As your aorta leaves the left ventricle, it passes upward (ascending aorta) before it begins to loop back down. The point at which the aorta turns is called the arch of the aorta, or aortic arch. The carotid arteries that pass through your neck and go up to the brain branch off from the aortic arch.

Arrhythmia: Arrhythmia is an irregularity in the rhythm or force of the heartbeat.

Arteriole: An arteriole is the smallest branch of an artery, which is in between the artery and the network of capillaries.

Artery: An artery is a muscular, flexible blood vessel that carries blood away from the heart and delivers it to the tissues of the body. Except for the pulmonary artery, which takes oxygen-poor blood from the heart to the lungs, arteries typically carry oxygen-rich blood.

Ascending aorta: The ascending aorta is that part of the aorta that passes upward toward the neck as it leaves the left ventricle of the heart.

Association neuron: Association neurons are found in the central nervous system (CNS). They act as bridges, carrying nerve impulses from sensory to motor neurons.

Asystole: Asystole literally means "without systole." Therefore, it is the absence of a heartbeat—failure of the ventricles of the heart to contract.

Atrial natriuretic peptide: Atrial natriuretic peptide (ANP) is a hormone that lowers blood pressure by causing vasodilation and by decreasing blood volume through promoting water and salt loss in urine.

Atrioventricular (AV) block: AV block (or heart block) refers to a blocking of the normal activity of the AV node, which results in nerve impulses either being slowed, partially skipped, or totally stopped from transmission to the ventricles.

Atrioventricular bundle: The AV bundle, or bundle of His, is a band of fibers in your heart through which impulses are transmitted from the AV node to the ventricles.

Atrioventricular node: The AV node (or sinus node) is an area of specialized heart muscle located in the wall of your right atrium. It receives impulses from the sinoatrial (SA) node, or the heart's internal pacemaker. Your AV node slows the impulses slightly before transmitting them to the AV bundle, which sends them to the ventricle wall.

Atrioventricular valves: There are two AV valves in your heart, each of which is located between an atrium and the ventricle beneath it. The tricuspid valve is located between your right atrium and ventricle; the bicuspid (or mitral) valve is between your left atrium and ventricle.

Atrium: (Plural is atria.) An atrium is either of the two smaller upper chambers of the heart. Your right atrium receives oxygen-poor blood from your systemic circulation and passes it into the right ventricle for transport to the lungs. Your left atrium receives oxygen-rich blood from the lungs and passes it into the left ventricle for circulation throughout the rest of your body.

Autonomic nervous system: Your ANS is that part of your peripheral nervous system (PNS) that automatically regulates involuntary functions of the body, such as heartbeat, breathing, sweating, temperature control, and digestion. It consists mostly of motor neurons, which carry nerve impulses from the CNS to different muscles and glands.

Autoregulation: Autoregulation is the process by which some internal mechanism detects and adjusts for changes within your system. In this instance, autoregulation refers to your body's automatic adjustment of blood flow to a particular tissue in response to the special needs of that tissue.

Axon: The axon is a long, thin extension of the cell body of a neuron, or nerve cell. Each neuron has only one axon. The axon receives nerve impulses from the cell body and transmits them to another neuron or to a tissue.

Axon terminals: Axon terminals are the many fine threadlike structures at the end of the axon on a neuron, or nerve cell.

Baroreceptor: Baroreceptors are structures in your body that are sensitive to changes in blood pressure. When your blood pressure is high, baroreceptors cause parasympathetic impulses, which are inhibitory, to be sent to the heart.

Beta-adrenergic receptors: Beta-adrenergic receptors are receptors that bind with epinephrine and other substances, allowing them to carry out their functions.

Beta-blocking agents: Beta-blocking agents lower blood pressure by blocking the stimulating effect of epinephrine on the heart, thereby reducing heart rate and the force of heart contractions.

Bicuspid valve: The bicuspid (or mitral) valve is the AV valve that allows blood to flow from the left atrium into the left ventricle of the heart. It is formed of two flaps, or cusps.

Biofeedback: Biofeedback is a training technique that enables you to gain some voluntary control over autonomic body functions, such as blood pressure.

Bipolar disorder: See manic-depressive disorder.

Blood–brain barrier: The blood–brain barrier is a mechanism that prevents the passage of certain materials from the blood into the brain and cerebrospinal fluid, which circulates around the brain and spinal cord.

Blood pressure: Blood pressure is the pressure that blood exerts on the inside wall of an artery. It is given as two measurements—systolic and diastolic blood pressures—expressed in millimeters of mercury (mm Hg). An example of a normal blood pressure reading is 120/80 mm Hg, in which 120 is the systolic reading and 80 is the diastolic reading.

Blood volume: Blood volume is the total amount of blood being circulated throughout your body at any one time—typically about 5 quarts.

Bradyarrhythmia: Bradyarrhythmia is a disturbance in the heart's normal rhythm that results in a slow heart rate.

Bradycardia: Bradycardia is a slow heart rate—usually under 60 beats per minute.

Brain: The brain, which is located in the skull, is the major organ of the nervous system. It is the body's control center, in addition to being the organ of human thought, speech, and emotion.

Brainstem: The brainstem is that part of the brain that is a continuation of the spinal cord. It consists of the medulla oblongata, pons, and midbrain. The brainstem is mainly concerned with the control of vital functions, such as breathing and blood pressure.

Bulimia: Bulimia is an eating disorder characterized by overeating (bingeing), followed by self-induced vomiting, fasting, or abuse of laxatives.

Bundle branches: Bundle branches are part of your heart's conduction system. Impulses pass from the AV node, to the AV bundle, and into the right and left bundle branches, which are located in the wall separating the two ventricles (interventricular septum). Actual contraction of the ventricle is stimulated by Purkinje fibers that emerge from the bundle branches.

Calcium channel–blocking agents: Calcium channel–blocking agents lower blood pressure by blocking the entry of calcium into smooth muscle, resulting in relaxation of heart muscle, dilation of heart and peripheral arteries, and slowing of heart rate.

Cancer: Cancer is a general term for various diseases characterized by uncontrolled growth and multiplication of abnormal cells, which tend to spread to other sites in the body (metastasize). Some cancers form solid masses of abnormal cells, called malignant tumors, that often invade surrounding tissues.

Capillaries: Capillaries are very tiny blood vessels that connect arterioles to venules. Thin capillary walls allow oxygen and nutrients to pass from oxygen-rich blood into body tissues. At the same time, carbon dioxide and other waste products pass out of tissues and into the capillary, which delivers the now oxygen-poor blood to the venules.

Carbohydrate: Carbohydrate is a general term that includes sugars, starches, and indigestible substances, such as fiber. Carbohydrates are a major source of energy.

Cardiac cycle: The cardiac cycle is the period from the beginning of one heartbeat to the beginning of the next.

Cardiac output: Cardiac output, which is the main factor in determining blood pressure, typically refers to the amount of blood your left ventricle ejects in a minute. To calculate cardiac output, multiply the amount of blood ejected during one contraction—stroke volume—by the number of heartbeats per minute.

Cardiopulmonary resuscitation (CPR): CPR is an emergency procedure used for a person who has collapsed, is unresponsive, has no pulse, and has stopped breathing. It consists of external heart massage and artificial respiration (maintaining airflow through the respiratory system).

Cardiovascular center: The cardiovascular center is a particular group of neurons, or nerve cells, located in your brain. The cardiovascular center affects heart rate, regulates how hard the heart contracts, and controls the diameter of blood vessels.

Cardiovascular system: Your cardiovascular system consists of your heart and various blood vessels—arteries, arterioles, capillaries, venules, and veins. The cardiovascular system is involved in the pumping of blood and the transport of oxygen and nutrients to cells and the removal of carbon dioxide and other waste products from cells.

Carotid sinus hypersensitivity: Carotid sinus hypersensitivity is an excessive response to pressure on the baroreceptors in the carotid sinus, resulting in slowing of heartbeat, reduced constriction of blood vessels, or a combination of the two—all of which can lower blood pressure.

Catecholamine: Catecholamine is a general term for neurotransmitters produced in your adrenal glands, including epinephrine, norepinephrine, and dopamine.

Cell body (of neuron): The cell body is one of three parts of a neuron, or nerve cell. (The other two parts are the axon and dendrites.) It is the larger central section from which the axon and dendrites extend.

Central nervous system: CNS consists of your brain and spinal cord.

Cerebellum: The cerebellum is the part of your brain located below the cerebrum and behind the brainstem. It is concerned mainly with the control of muscular coordination, balance, and posture.

Cerebral cortex: The cerebral cortex is the thin, heavily folded layer of gray matter on the surface of the cerebrum portion of your brain. The cerebral cortex is the center for higher mental functions, perception, and behavioral responses, among other functions.

Cerebrovascular disease: Cerebrovascular disease is a general term that includes any conditions that can cause a stroke due to hemorrhage or blockage of an artery in the brain.

Cerebrovascular system: Your cerebrovascular system refers to the blood vessels carrying oxygen and nutrients to and removing carbon dioxide and other waste products from your brain. The circulation of blood in your brain is sometimes called cerebral circulation.

Cerebrum: The cerebrum is the part of the brain that spreads over the diencephalon, filling much of the skull (or cranium). It has two sides, called hemispheres. The outer surface of the cerebrum, the cerebral cortex, is concerned with conscious thought, movement, and sensation.

Cervical nerves: Your cervical nerves are the eight pairs of nerves originating in the spinal cord at the level of your neck.

Chemoreceptors: Chemoreceptors are special nerve cells (neurons) that are sensitive to chemical substances in the blood. They respond to abnormally low levels of oxygen and higher than normal levels of carbon dioxide and hydrogen in the blood by sending impulses to the vasomotor center of the brain. The vasomotor center increases sympathetic stimulation of the arterioles, resulting in vasoconstriction and an increase in blood pressure.

Chronic fatigue syndrome (CFS): CFS is characterized by chronic, debilitating fatigue. Other symptoms may include difficulty in short-term memory or concentration, sore throat, tender lymph nodes in the neck or armpits, muscle pain, pain that moves from one joint to another (with no redness or swelling), headaches with a new pattern or severity, sleep that does not make you feel rested, and/or fatigue lasting 24 hours or more following exercise that you previously have tolerated.

Clonic: Clonic refers to alternating contraction and relaxation of a muscle.

Clonidine: Clonidine is a drug that acts as an alpha-2-adrenergic agonist, that is, it inhibits the outflow of sympathetic impulses.

Coccygeal nerves: Coccygeal nerves are the one pair of nerves originating in your spinal cord at the very bottom of your spinal column—your "tailbone."

Collagen: Collagen is a protein that is the main organic component of connective tissue.

Congestive heart failure: Congestive heart failure (or heart failure) is a condition caused by the inability of the heart to circulate an adequate amount of blood to the lungs and other tissues in the body. Symptoms typically include shortness of breath, weakness, and edema (excessive fluid build-up in tissues).

Constrictive pericarditis: Pericarditis is an inflammation of the loose-fitting sac (pericardium) enclosing the heart. Constrictive pericarditis occurs when the inflammation causes a build-up of blood or fluid in the space between the heart and the pericardium, putting pressure on the heart and making it unable to function properly.

Convulsion: A convulsion is an intensive, sudden, involuntary muscular contraction.

Coronary arteries: You have two coronary arteries, which branch off from the aorta and supply blood to the heart itself.

Coronary artery disease: Coronary artery disease refers to the gradual blocking of the arteries in the heart by the build-up of material, called plaque, in and on the surface of the artery walls.

Deep vein thrombosis: Deep vein thrombosis is the formation of a blood clot in veins that are located deep in the leg, pelvis, or even arm.

Defibrillator: A defibrillator is an electronic device used to apply electrical shocks to the heart. It is used to restore normal heart rhythm in people experiencing ventricular tachycardia (V-tach, or VT) or ventricular fibrillation.

Dehydration: Dehydration refers to a large loss of water from your body.

Dementia: Dementia is a progressive deterioration of intellectual faculties, including memory, concentration, and judgment.

Dendrite: A dendrite is one of several short, thick, and highly branched extensions from the cell body of a neuron, or nerve cell. It receives incoming nerve impulses from either a sensory receptor or another nerve cell and then transmits it to the cell body.

Depression: Depression is a state of mind characterized by sadness, discouragement, and hopelessness, often accompanied by reduced activity and ability to function, unresponsiveness, and sleep disturbances, among other symptoms. A continuing sad mood—being "down in the dumps" most of the time—is known as dysthymia. Major depression is a more serious form of depression, which sometimes ends in suicide.

Diabetes insipidus: Diabetes insipidus is a condition caused by too little antidiuretic hormone (ADH) (or vasopressin) being secreted. It results in thirst and excretion of large amounts of urine.

Diabetes mellitus: Diabetes mellitus is a chronic metabolic disease in which the hormone insulin is either not produced or not effective in transporting glucose from blood to the body's cells. This results in abnormally high blood glucose levels and increased urination and thirst, among other symptoms.

Diabetic neuropathy: Diabetic neuropathy is a condition in which diabetes mellitus results in damage to neurons (nerve cells) in peripheral nerves. Diabetic neuropathy can include damage to sensory, motor, autonomic, or all three types of neurons.

Diaphragm: Your diaphragm is a dome-shaped muscle stretching across the inside of your body and separating your chest from your abdomen. It moves downward when you breathe in (inhale) to increase the volume of your chest and moves upward when you breathe out (exhale).

Diastole: Diastole is the period between two heart contractions—the relaxation phase. During diastole the chambers of the heart fill with blood.

Diastolic blood pressure: Diastolic blood pressure is a measurement of the remaining force exerted against artery walls during diastole, when the heart muscle is relaxed. In a normal blood pressure reading, such as 120/80 mm Hg, 80 is the diastolic measurement.

Diencephalon: The diencephalon is the area of the brain located above your brainstem. It consists primarily of two glands: the thalamus and the hypothalamus.

Digitalis: Digitalis is a heart stimulant used in the treatment of congestive heart failure and other heart disorders.

Disopyramide: Disopyramide is a heart suppressant that is used to prevent arrhythmia, or an irregular heart rhythm.

Diuretic: A diuretic is any substance that increases the amount of fluid excreted through your kidneys in urine.

Dopamine: Dopamine is a neurotransmitter in the CNS and also acts on receptors in blood vessels. It usually excites a response instead of inhibiting it. Decreased levels of dopamine are associated with Parkinson's disease.

Dopamine-β-hydroxylase deficiency: This condition is a deficiency of dopamine-β-hydroxylase, which is the enzyme that aids in the conversion of dopamine to norepinephrine.

Double-blind study: A double-blind study is one in which neither participants nor staff members know whether a particular participant is assigned to the treatment group(s) or to a control group.

Drop attack: A drop attack refers to suddenly losing consciousness without first experiencing any warning symptoms.

Dysautonomic: The term dysautonomic indicates abnormal functioning of the ANS.

Efferent neuron: See motor neuron.

Electrocardiogram (ECG, or EKG): An ECG is a test in which the electrical activity of your heart is recorded.

Electroencephalogram (EEG): An EEG is a test in which the electrical activity of your brain is recorded.

Electrophysiological (EP) testing: EP testing is used to evaluate various arrhythmias.

Endless-loop recorder: An endless-loop (or event) recorder is a portable electrocardiograph machine that continuously records the electrical activity of the heart over extended periods of time.

Endocardium: The endocardium is the membrane that lines the inside of the heart chambers and covers the heart valves.

Endocrine system: The endocrine system consists of a number of glands (pituitary, thyroid, parathyroid, adrenal, pineal, and thymus) and other tissues that secrete hormones and pass them directly into the bloodstream.

Endothelium: The endothelium is a layer of cells that lines your heart, blood vessels, lymph vessels, and some body cavities.

Enzyme: An enzyme is a substance that affects the speed of a chemical change. Several enzymes are important in blood pressure control.

Ephedrine: Ephedrine is a drug used primarily in the treatment of asthma and allergies.

Epicardium: The epicardium is the thin layer of membrane covering the outside of your heart.

Epilepsy: Epilepsy is a disorder of the nervous system that is characterized by sudden, recurring attacks of motor, sensory, or psychic malfunction. Epilepsy can occur with or without convulsive seizures and/or loss of consciousness.

Epinephrine: Epinephrine (or adrenaline) is a hormone secreted by your adrenal glands. It produces activities that facilitate sympathetic activity, including regulating blood vessels, strengthening heart contractions, and increasing heart, breathing, and metabolic rates. Epinephrine acts as a powerful stimulant in times of fear or arousal—the fight or flight response.

Erythropoietin: Erythropoietin is a hormone involved in the control of red cell production for your blood. It is sometimes used to treat people who faint because of anemia.

Excitability (of a nerve): A nerve's degree of "excitability" is its ability to respond to a stimulus and to convert it into a nerve impulse.

Fludrocortisone: Fludrocortisone is a mineralocorticoid drug that increases blood pressure by expanding blood volume and making your blood vessels more sensitive to the constrictive effects of norepinephrine.

Ganglion: A ganglion is a small knot or group of nerve cells that lies outside the CNS. (The plural form of ganglion is usually ganglia.)

Glucose: Glucose is a simple sugar that is the primary fuel source for the human body. Your blood carries glucose to all the cells of your body, leading to its being called "blood sugar."

Guillain-Barré syndrome: Guillain-Barré syndrome is a type of rapidly progressive inflammation of the peripheral nerves. It results in pain and weakness and sometimes may cause paralysis of the limbs.

Heart murmur: A heart murmur is an abnormal sound heard during the heartbeat.

Hemoglobin count: A hemoglobin count is a measurement of the oxygen-carrying component in red blood cells.

Hemorrhage: Hemorrhage is any excessive loss of blood from your blood vessels in a short amount of time. A hemorrhage can be internal or external.

Hepatic circulation: Hepatic circulation refers to that part of systemic circulation that circulates blood in your liver.

Hepatitis: Hepatitis is an inflammation of the liver. It is usually accompanied by jaundice (yellow color of the skin), loss of appetite, abdominal discomfort, an enlarged liver that is functioning abnormally, and dark urine.

Holter monitor: A Holter monitor is a portable electrocardiogram that records your heart's electrical activity as you go about your daily activities.

Homeostasis: Homeostasis is the condition in which your body's internal environment remains relatively constant, that is, within a certain range. The body automatically adjusts to different internal processes to maintain this balance.

Hormone: A hormone is a substance produced by one tissue in your body and carried by the bloodstream to target tissues or organs, where it alters the physiological activity. Several hormones are important in blood pressure control.

HIV: Infection with the HIV causes acquired immunodeficiency syndrome (AIDS).

Huntington's disease: Huntington's disease (or Huntington's chorea or hereditary chorea) is an inherited chronic disorder characterized by involuntary spasmodic twitching or jerking in muscle groups of the face and extremities, accompanied by a gradual loss of mental faculties ending in dementia.

Hypertension: Hypertension is persistent high blood pressure. It is defined as a systolic blood pressure of 140 mm Hg or greater and diastolic blood pressure of 90 mm Hg or greater.

Hyperventilation: Hyperventilation is abnormally fast and/or deep breathing that causes a loss of carbon dioxide from the blood, which may result in a loss of blood pressure and fainting.

Hypoglycemia: Hypoglycemia is an abnormally low level of the sugar glucose in the blood. It can cause symptoms such as dizziness, confusion, convulsions, and/or a loss of consciousness.

Hypokalemia: Hypokalemia is a low level of potassium in the blood.

Hypopituitarism: Hypopituitarism is an underactive pituitary gland.

Hypotension: Hypotension is low blood pressure, usually a systolic reading of 90 mm Hg or less. The term is often used to describe a rapid drop in blood pressure, such as can occur in shock and certain other situations.

Hypothalamus: The hypothalamus is known as the body's "master gland" because it controls so many activities. For example, the hypothalamus controls and organizes the activities of the ANS and regulates the release of many hormones from the pituitary gland.

Hypothyroidism: Hypothyroidism is a decreased activity of the thyroid gland, which can result in fatigue, lack of energy, sensitivity to cold, and weight gain, among other signs and symptoms.

Hypoxia: Hypoxia is a low level of oxygen in the blood or body tissues.

Impotence: Impotence is the condition of being incapable of sexual intercourse, often because of an inability to achieve or sustain an erection.

Incontinence: In this instance, incontinence refers to a lack of bladder and bowel control.

Integration function: The nervous system's integration function is the analysis of information gained in its sensory function. The information is then either stored or goes to the nervous system's motor function, which initiates action.

Interatrial septum: The interatrial septum is the wall between the two atria of the heart.

Interventricular septum: The interventricular septum is the wall between the two ventricles of the heart.

Intravenous (IV): IV refers to something within or administered into a vein.

Isometrically: Isometrically refers to contracting a muscle without shortening its length.

Jet lag: Jet lag is a temporary disturbance of normal circadian rhythm—your biological clock, which governs your wake-sleep cycle. It is caused by high-speed travel across several time zones, usually in a jet aircraft. Jet lag usually causes fatigue, sleep disturbances, and sluggish body functions.

Kidneys: Your kidneys are two bean-shaped organs that filter wastes from the blood and excrete them with water in urine.

Lumbar nerves: Lumbar nerves are the five pairs of nerves originating in your spinal cord at the level of the lower back.

Lumen: The lumen is the interior space of a tubelike structure, such as a blood vessel.

Lupus: See systemic lupus erythematosus.

Manic-depressive disorder: Manic-depressive (or bipolar) disorder is characterized by periodic swings from mania (euphoria, many rapidly changing ideas, exaggerated gaiety, and excessive physical activity) to depression.

Mechanoreceptors: Mechanoreceptors are receptors found in the atria and ventricles of your heart and in the pulmonary arteries leading to the lungs. They are sensitive to being stretched, as when the heart chambers fill with blood.

Methyldopa: Methyldopa is a drug used in the treatment of high blood pressure.

Methylphenidate: Methylphenidate is a drug that stimulates the CNS, causes vasoconstriction, and increases the release of dopamine and norepinephrine (neurotransmitters) in the part of the nervous system that affects body posture and reflex mechanisms.

Midodrine: Midodrine, which is the only drug approved by the U.S. Food and Drug Administration for the treatment of orthostatic hypotension, is also used to treat neurocardiogenic syncope and postural tachycardia syndrome (POTS). This alpha-1 agonist increases blood pressure by constricting blood vessels.

Milking: Milking is a term used to describe how alternating contraction and relaxation of skeletal muscles can help move blood from the lower body back toward the heart.

Mitral valve: The mitral (or bicuspid) valve is an AV valve that allows blood to flow from the left atrium into the left ventricle of the heart. It is formed of two flaps, or cusps.

Mitral valve prolapse: Mitral valve prolapse is an inherited disorder in which part of the mitral valve is pushed back too far (prolapsed) during the contraction of the left ventricle, allowing a small amount of blood to flow back into the left atrium.

Motor function: The nervous system's motor function refers to the action that results from information gained in its sensory function and analyzed in its integration function. In its motor function, the nervous system responds to stimuli by initiating action—contracting your muscles or causing your glands to produce and release substances such as hormones.

Motor neurons: Motor (or efferent) neurons are specialized nerve cells that start in the CNS and carry nerve impulses to the muscles and glands that are targeted by the motor functions of the nervous system. Basically, they handle outgoing orders.

Multiple sclerosis: Multiple sclerosis is a progressive disease, usually starting in early adulthood, in which the axons of nerve fibers in the brain and spinal cord lose their protective myelin cover.

Multiple system atrophy: Multiple system atrophy consists of several over-lapping syndromes. In addition to the orthostatic hypotension, impotence, bladder dysfunction, and defective-sweating characteristic of pure autonomic failure, people with multiple system atrophy also have symptoms such as rigidity and tremor, among others. The best known type of multiple system atrophy is Shy-Drager syndrome.

Myocardial infarction (MI): MI is a heart attack. It is the death of an area of heart muscle resulting from an interruption of the blood supply due to a blocked artery.

Myocarditis: Myocarditis is an inflammation of the myocardium (muscular middle layer) of the heart.

Myocardium: The myocardium is the thick, muscular middle layer of the heart wall. It consists of thick bundles of special cardiac muscle that do not occur anywhere else in the body.

Narcolepsy: Narcolepsy is a disorder characterized by sudden, uncontrollable, usually brief attacks of deep sleep.

Neurocardiogenic syncope: Neurocardiogenic (or vasovagal) syncope is a temporary loss of consciousness associated with a drop in arterial blood pressure, quickly followed by a slowed heart rate (bradycardia). It is thought to be due to mechanoreceptors (receptors that respond to being stretched) in the heart misinterpreting the drop in blood pressure and sending the ANS messages that indicate the opposite condition—high blood pressure.

Neuroglandular junction: The neuroglandular junction is the tiny space that separates the axon of a postganglionic neuron (between a ganglion and target organ) and the gland it stimulates.

Neuromuscular junction: The neuromuscular junction is the tiny space that separates the axon of a postganglionic neuron (between a ganglion and target organ) and the muscle cell it stimulates.

Neuron: Neuron is the technical name for a nerve cell. It has three parts: the cell body, an axon, and dendrites.

Neurotransmitter: Neurotransmitters are chemical substances synthesized in the axon terminals of nerve cells and released into the synapse in response to a nerve impulse. Neurotransmitters act on the receptors located on the dendrites of the next neuron (postsynaptic neuron), muscle fibers (at neuromuscular junction), or cells in glands (at neuroglandular junction). Neurotransmitters can transmit one of two types of impulses. Excitatory transmissions create a new nerve impulse, which continues the original impulse. Inhibitory transmissions prevent the nerve impulse from continuing.

Norepinephrine: Norepinephrine (or noradrenaline) is a hormone neurotransmitter found in the CNS. It can be excitatory or inhibitory and facilitates sympathetic activity. Its activities include constricting blood vessels, slowing heart rate, increasing breathing rate, and raising blood pressure, among others.

Orthostatic hypotension: Orthostatic (or postural) hypotension is an excessive lowering of systemic blood pressure when you assume an erect or partially erect posture. It can be caused by excessive fluid loss, certain drugs, and factors associated with the cardiovascular or nervous systems.

Orthostatic intolerance: Orthostatic intolerance is an inability to move to an upright position without experiencing symptoms.

Otolaryngologist: An otolaryngologist is a doctor who specializes in evaluating and treating conditions of the ear, nose, and throat.

Pacing: Pacing is the insertion of an artificial pacemaker to stimulate or regulate the heart's contractions.

Pallor: Pallor is abnormal paleness of the skin.

Palpitations: Palpitations are the feeling that the heart is beating rapidly and forcefully or fluttering. Palpitations are often associated with strong emotions or with certain abnormalities of the heart.

Panic disorder: Panic disorder is a psychiatric condition characterized by recurring intense attacks of anxiety in specific circumstances and situations. Symptoms typically include shortness of breath, pounding and/or racing heart, chest pain, sweating, dizziness, trembling or shaking, and fear of dying or of losing mental functioning (going "crazy"), among others.

Parasympathetic division: The parasympathetic division is one of the two subdivisions of the ANS (the other being the sympathetic division). It is concerned primarily with processes that save and restore energy in the body.

Parkinson's disease: Parkinson's disease (or parkinsonism) is a slowly progressive disorder of the nervous system. It is associated with a decreased production of dopamine, which leads to tremor, slowing of voluntary movements, and muscle weakness.

Peripheral nervous system: The PNS consists of the nerves that arise from the brain and spinal cord. These nerves carry nerve impulses both into and out of the CNS.

Peripheral resistance: Peripheral resistance is the opposition to the flow of blood vessels that results from friction between blood and blood vessel walls. Larger blood vessels have lower peripheral resistance than smaller vessels. The ability of arterioles to change peripheral resistance is an important factor in the regulation of blood pressure.

Placebo-controlled study: A placebo-controlled study is one in which one group receives an inactive substance or preparation—a placebo—that resembles the drug under investigation. Researchers compare the results observed in participants taking the drug to those of participants taking the placebo in order to determine the effectiveness of or to test the drug.

Polyneuropathy: Polyneuropathy refers to a generalized disorder of the peripheral nerves.

Porphyria: Porphyria is any of several inherited disorders in which large amounts of metal-containing compounds, called porphyrins, are found in blood and urine.

Postganglionic neuron: A postganglionic neuron is a nerve cell located between the ganglion (knot of nerve cells in the PNS) and the muscle or gland to which it carries nerve impulses.

Postprandial hypotension: Postprandial hypotension is a decrease in systolic blood pressure of 20 mm Hg or more within 2 hours of starting a meal.

Postsyncope: Postsyncope refers to the period immediately after someone who has fainted regains consciousness.

Postural tachycardia syndrome: POTS consists of a very fast heart rate—tachycardia—that occurs after you stand up. POTS is defined as the development of orthostatic symptoms due to an increase in heart rate of at least 30 beats per minute or a heart rate of at least 120 beats per minute occurring within the first 10 minutes of standing. This condition is sometimes, but not always, associated with mild low blood pressure.

Preganglionic neuron: A preganglionic neuron is a nerve cell located between the brain or spinal cord and the ganglion, which is a knot of nerve cells in the PNS.

Presyncope: Presyncope refers to the symptoms typically preceding a faint.

Provocation agent: A provocation agent is a drug with effects similar to epinephrine (adrenaline). It increases your heart rate and helps show what occurs when your heart is beating faster. The most commonly used provocation agent is isoproterenol; others include nitroglycerin, edrophonium, adenosine triphosphate, epinephrine, and nitroprusside.

Pseudoephedrine: Pseudoephedrine is an adrenergic agent used primarily as a nasal decongestant in both prescription and over-the-counter products.

Pulmonary artery: The pulmonary artery carries oxygen-poor blood from the right ventricle of the heart to the lungs where it can pick up oxygen.

Pulmonary circulation: Pulmonary circulation refers to the blood vessels carrying blood to and from your heart to your lungs.

Pulmonary embolism: A pulmonary embolism is a blockage of an artery in the lung by a blood clot that was formed elsewhere in the body.

Pulmonary vein: There are two pulmonary veins, one leaving each lung, that carry oxygen-rich blood from the lungs back to the left atrium of the heart.

Pure autonomic failure: This disorder of the ANS is characterized by orthostatic hypotension, impotence, bladder dysfunction, and defective sweating.

Purkinje fibers: Purkinje fibers are tiny specialized muscle fibers that emerge from the right and left bundle branches located in the wall separating the two ventricles of the heart. Purkinje fibers distribute the impulse that originated in the SA node to the cells in the ventricle's muscular middle layer (myocardium), causing them to contract.

Randomized study: A randomized study is one in which study participants are assigned to different treatment groups according to some known probability distribution. Randomization is used to prevent bias in studies.

Renin: Renin is an enzyme secreted by the kidneys in response to a decrease in blood pressure. Renin raises blood pressure by influencing your kidneys to retain fluid, which increases blood volume, and by causing vasoconstriction.

Sacral nerves: Sacral nerves are the five pairs of nerves originating in your spinal cord at the level of the pelvis, where the spine connects with the legs.

Schizophrenia: Schizophrenia refers to a group of mental disorders characterized by withdrawal from reality, illogical patterns of thinking, hallucinations, delusions, and withdrawal from social contacts, among other symptoms.

Sedative: In this instance, sedative refers to a drug that produces a soothing, calming, or tranquilizing effect.

Seizure: A seizure is a sudden attack, spasm, or convulsion, as in epilepsy.

Selective serotonin reuptake inhibitor (SSRI): SSRIs are agents that inhibit the reuptake of serotonin by its receptors, resulting in larger amounts of serotonin remaining in the synapse between nerve cells (neurons). SSRIs are typically used as antidepressants.

Semilunar valves: The heart's semilunar valves, which are shaped somewhat like a half moon, prevent blood that is being pumped out of the heart and into the arteries from flowing backward into the ventricles.

Sensory function: In its sensory (or afferent) function, your nervous system senses changes inside and outside your body.

Sensory neuron: Sensory (or afferent) neurons are specialized nerve cells that carry impulses from the sensory receptors to the CNS. Basically, they handle incoming information.

Sepsis: Sepsis is an infection of a wound or tissue caused by bacteria and leading to the formation of pus. It is often accompanied by a fever. Sepsis can also mean the presence of pathogenic organisms in your blood.

Serotonin: Serotonin is a neurotransmitter found in the CNS. It typically acts to inhibit the transmission of nerve impulses.

Shy-Drager syndrome: Shy-Drager syndrome is a severe form of multiple system atrophy that is accompanied by failure of the ANS.

Sick sinus syndrome: Sick sinus syndrome results from malfunctions of the sinus (or AV) node. It may include both bradyarrhythmia (irregular slow heart rate) and tachyarrhythmia (irregular fast heart rate), which can cause the symptoms preceding a faint.

Sinoatrial node: The SA node is an area of specialized heart muscle in the right atrium. The SA node, which is called the heart's pacemaker, initiates impulses that travel through the muscles of both atria, causing them to contract. Cells in the SA node have a rhythm that is independent of the nervous system.

Skeletal muscle: Skeletal muscle is a type of muscle that specializes in contraction. Skeletal muscles are attached to bones and are stimulated to move the bones by motor neurons of the somatic nervous system.

Sleep apnea: Sleep apnea is a temporary stoppage of breathing while asleep.

Sodium: Sodium is a metal that is very important for human health. Its vital functions are its roles in water balance, nerve transmission, and muscle contraction, among others.

Somatic nervous system: Your PNS has two parts: somatic and ANS. Your somatic nervous system controls conscious responses and movements. Its sensory neurons pick up information from your head, trunk, arms, and legs and send it to the CNS. Its motor neurons carry nerve impulses only to your skeletal muscles, where they cause muscles to contract.

Somatization: Somatization is a condition in which a person reports many physical symptoms, usually involving a variety of organ systems, for which the doctor can find no physical cause.

Spinal cord: The spinal cord is a mass of nerve tissue running down the canal in your spine. It is the origin of 31 pairs of spinal nerves. The spinal cord and brain make up the CNS.

Spinal nerve: The term spinal nerve refers to one of the 31 pairs of nerves originating in the spinal cord.

Stimulus: A stimulus is a "stress" or change inside or outside the body that excites a nerve or muscle fiber. In this instance, a stimulus usually refers to anything in the internal or external environment that can cause a neuron that is not carrying a nerve impulse to change its electrical charge so that it is able to carry the impulse.

Stroke: A stroke (or cerebrovascular accident) is a potentially fatal loss of brain function caused by a lack of oxygen to brain cells due to hemorrhage or blockage of blood vessels in the brain. Symptoms may include weakness, a sudden loss of muscular control, dizziness, slurred speech or an inability to speak, and/or paralysis.

Stroke volume: Stroke volume refers to the amount of blood ejected during one contraction of the heart.

Subdural hematoma: A subdural hematoma is a leakage of blood in the brain.

Sudden infant death syndrome (SIDS): SIDS is a fatal syndrome affecting apparently healthy babies less than 1 year old, who suddenly stop breathing while asleep.

Supine hypertension: Supine refers to lying on your back. Supine hypertension is high blood pressure that occurs when you are lying down.

Sympathetic division: The sympathetic division is one of the two subdivisions of the ANS (the other being the parasympathetic division). It is primarily concerned with processes that use, or expend, energy.

Synapse: A synapse is the tiny space between the axon of one neuron and the dendrites of the next one in line.

Synaptic end bulbs: Synaptic end bulbs are bulblike structures at the end of axon terminals that are threadlike structures at the end of the axon on a neuron, or nerve cell. Synaptic end bulbs contain sacs (synaptic vesicles) that store neurotransmitters.

Synaptic vesicles: Synaptic vesicles are sacs that store neurotransmitters, which are chemical substances that transmit nerve impulses across the synapse between neurons, or nerve cells. Synaptic vesicles are located in the synaptic end bulbs at the end of the axon terminals—the threadlike structures at the end of the axon on a neuron.

Syncope: Syncope is a temporary loss of consciousness—a faint. One common cause of syncope is insufficient blood supply to the brain.

Syringomyelia: Syringomyelia is a progressive disease of the spinal cord in which the tissue develops holes surrounded by scar tissue. Symptoms include sensory loss, weakness, and muscle atrophy (decrease in size from wasting).

Systemic circulation: Systemic circulation refers to the blood vessels transporting blood to and from your heart to all the parts of your body, with the exception of your lungs.

Systemic lupus erythematosus: Systemic lupus erythematosus ("lupus") is a chronic inflammatory disease affecting many body systems, which occurs more often in women. Symptoms include fever, weakness, being easily fatigued, joint pains or arthritis, and a red "butterfly" rash over the nose and cheeks, among others.

Systole: Systole refers to the contraction of the heart, especially the ventricles. When the right ventricle contracts, blood is pumped out of the heart and into the pulmonary artery to go to the lungs. Contraction of the more muscular left ventricle ejects blood into the aorta to be carried to the rest of the body.

Systolic blood pressure: Systolic blood pressure is a measurement of the force of blood pressing outward on the artery wall during systole, when the heart is contracting. In a normal blood pressure reading, such as 120/80 mm Hg, 120 is the systolic measurement.

Tabes dorsalis: Tabes dorsalis is an abnormal condition that is characterized by a progressive degeneration of sensory neurons. Symptoms usually include severe stabbing pains in the legs and trunk of the body, unsteady gait, defective reflexes, incontinence, and impotence. Tabes dorsalis typically occurs 15–20 years after an initial infection with syphilis (a sexually transmitted disease).

Tachyarrhythmia: Tachyarrhythmia is a heartbeat that is both rapid and irregular, causing a reduction in normal blood flow from the heart to the rest of the body.

Tachycardia: Tachycardia is a rapid heart rate, that is, a heart rate above 100 beats per minute (in an adult).

Theophylline: Theophylline is a bronchodilator, that is, a drug that opens bronchial air passages (main branches of the windpipe, leading into the lungs). Theophylline is used primarily to treat bronchial asthma and other lung conditions.

Thoracic aorta: The thoracic aorta is the portion of the descending aorta that is the origin of arteries in the chest area.

Thoracic nerves: The thoracic nerves are 12 pairs of nerves originating in the spinal cord at the level of the chest.

Tilt-table test: A tilt-table test mimics your body's responses when you stand up from a lying position, allowing the doctor to see what happens when your body is tilted—head up—from a horizontal position.

Tonic: In this instance, tonic refers to a sustained muscle contraction.

Transient ischemic attack (TIA): A TIA is a brief blockage of the blood supply to an area of the brain, usually caused by a blood clot. Symptoms may include dizziness, blurred vision, and numbness on one side of the body, among others. It is sometimes called a "mini-stroke."

Transverse myelitis: Transverse myelitis is an inflammation of the spinal cord affecting the entire width of the cord at a given level.

Tremulousness: Tremulousness refers to trembling, quivering, and feeling shaky.

Tricuspid valve: The tricuspid valve is the AV valve that allows blood to flow from the right atrium into the right ventricle of the heart. It is formed of three flaps, or cusps.

Tunica externa: The tunica externa, or "outer coat," is the outer layer of arteries and veins.

Tunica intima: The tunica intima, or "inner coat," is the inner layer of arteries and veins. In veins, this layer folds to form valves, which play an important role in returning blood to the heart.

Tunica media: The tunica media, or "middle coat," is the middle layer of arteries and veins. This layer, which consists of smooth muscle and elastic tissue, is much thicker in arteries than in veins.

"Tunnel" vision: Tunnel vision means that you can see things directly in front of you—in a narrow tunnel—but not off to the side.

Valsalva maneuver: The Valsalva maneuver is similar to "popping your ears" in an airplane. It is the effort to exhale when the mouth is closed and the nose is pinched shut. This forces air into the eustachian tubes that run between the back of the throat and the ear and increases pressure on the inside of the eardrum.

Vasoconstriction: Vasoconstriction is a decrease in the size of the space inside a blood vessel (lumen) caused by contraction of the smooth muscle in the vessel wall.

Vasodilation: Vasodilation is an increase in the size of the lumen of a blood vessel caused by relaxation of the smooth muscle in the vessel wall.

Vasomotor center: The vasomotor center is a cluster of nerve cells (neurons) in the brain that are part of the sympathetic division of the ANS. By controlling lumen (hollow opening inside a blood vessel) size, especially in the arterioles located in the skin and abdomen, the vasomotor center acts as the integrating center for blood pressure control.

Vasopressin: Vasopressin is an ADH, that is, it prevents too much urine from being excreted.

Vasovagal syncope: See neurocardiogenic syncope.

Vein: Veins are blood vessels that carry blood to the heart. With the exception of the pulmonary vein, which transports oxygen-rich blood from the lungs to the heart, veins typically carry oxygen-poor blood to the heart. Veins are less muscular than arteries and have valves to aid in returning blood to the heart.

Vena cava: A vena cava is either of two large veins that return oxygen-poor blood to the right atrium of the heart. The superior (higher) vena cava returns blood from the head, neck, chest, and arms. The inferior (lower) vena cava returns blood from the parts of the body below the diaphragm.

Ventricle: A ventricle is either of the two lower chambers of the heart. Ventricles are larger and more muscular than atria. The right ventricle receives oxygen-poor blood from the right atrium and pumps it to the lungs. The left ventricle receives oxygen-rich blood from the left atrium and pumps it throughout the body (except for the lungs). Because it must pump blood to a much larger area, the left ventricle has thicker, more muscular walls than the right ventricle.

Ventricular fibrillation: Ventricular fibrillation is a type of arrhythmia (irregular heartbeat) that is sometimes fatal. It consists of a rapid, disorganized twitching of individual muscle fibers in which the muscular wall of the ventricle is unable to contract as a whole, resulting in a loss of heartbeat.

Ventricular tachycardia: V-tach (or VT) is three or more consecutive ventricular premature beats. The rate is elevated to 160–240 beats per minute. The rapid heartbeat does not allow the heart to pump blood properly, potentially leading to cardiac arrest and death.

Venule: Venules are small veins. They extend from a capillary network and merge together to form a vein.

Vertigo: Vertigo is a sensation that either you or the things around you are revolving or spinning.

Yohimbine: Yohimbine is a drug that helps sympathetic impulses increase vasoconstriction. It increases blood pressure by causing a small increase in blood norepinephrine levels.

Index

Note: page numbers in *italics* refer to figures, those in **bold** refer to tables.